Extended Matching Items
for the
MRCPsych Part 1

Michael Reilly
MRCPsych, DipMang
Senior Registrar
University College Hospital, Galway, Ireland

Bangaru Raju
MD, MRCPsych, DPM
Senior Registrar
Area 6 Psychiatric Services, Dublin North West, Ireland

Radcliffe Publishing
Oxford • San Francisco

Radcliffe Publishing Ltd
18 Marcham Road
Abingdon
Oxon OX14 1AA
United Kingdom

www.radcliffe-oxford.com
Electronic catalogue and worldwide online ordering facility.

British Library Cataloguing in Publication Data

A catalogue record for this book is available from the British Library.

ISBN 1 85775 672 X

Typeset by Richard Powell Editorial and Production Services, Basingstoke, Hants
Printed and bound by TJ International Ltd, Padstow, Cornwall

Dedication

We dedicate this book to our children:

To Nicole,
and to Dhivya and Deepa
and any yet to arrive.

Contents

Introduction   *v*
Acknowledgements   *ix*
Instructions for Readers   *x*

EMIs

Psychology and Human Development EMIs   1
Psychopharmacology EMIs   41
Descriptive and Psychodynamic Psychopathology EMIs   79
Clinical Theory and Skills EMIs   117

Answers to EMIs

Psychology and Human Development EMIs   163
Psychopharmacology EMIs   174
Descriptive and Psychodynamic Psychopathology EMIs   184
Clinical Theory and Skills EMIs   194

References   209
Index of Questions   211

Introduction

> *If you know the enemy and know yourself,*
> *you need not fear the result of a hundred*
> *battles.*
>
> Sun-Tzu, *The Art of War*

Extended matching items (EMIs) were introduced to the MRCPsych written examinations in 2003. Educationalists prefer the use of multiple choice questions (MCQs) that have many items to choose from, since such questions tend to discriminate better between candidates of varying ability and are less 'guessable'[1]. The individual statements that currently make up the bulk of the questions on the MCQ papers are thus not optimal for examination purposes, especially as one has a 50% chance of guessing any given question correctly. The College is likely, therefore, to gradually reduce the proportion of individual statement-type questions and increase the proportion of EMIs on the paper over time (at the time of writing, the proportions are roughly 4-to-1, respectively).

One factor that will slow this transition, however, is the difficulty in producing a sufficient bank of EMIs. There has been relatively little experience with the format in either undergraduate or postgraduate examinations in psychiatry to date in Ireland or Great Britain. In addition, this format of question is quite difficult to compose if one wishes to avoid flaws that can aid the test-wise candidate. These factors are likely to mean that the individual statement type of question will continue to appear on the MRCPsych MCQ papers for the foreseeable future. They also mean, however, that there will likely be a dearth of material to help candidates prepare for the EMIs for some time. It was the latter realisation, together with the authors' observation of the anxiety this new question format was having on many trainees, which led to the conception of this book.

EMIs have four main elements[2]. The *theme* sets the scene and allows the candidate to develop an appropriate mental 'set' for the questions to follow. The *options list* varies in number from three to twenty-six concepts or short phrases, arranged alphabetically and each denoted by a letter of the alphabet. The *lead-in* gives instructions as to what is required from candidates in answering the questions. The questions themselves are termed *stems*, and there are at least two of these in each EMI.

The Royal College of Psychiatrists has provided three sample EMIs on its website[3]. Analysis of these, together with feedback from the first cohort of candidates who experienced the EMIs, suggests the College will mainly employ EMIs with ten options and three stems. Some of these stems will require candidates to select more than one option in answering. A number of these trainees, however, have noted that the EMIs that have appeared in the examination have been considerably more challenging than the samples and that the format was altered to a degree in some of these.

Despite the relative paucity of information on the EMIs, the authors have tried to produce questions that resemble those set by the College to allow candidates to become familiarised with this new part of the examination. However, given that these questions can have a number of variations in format (and that the College appears to be experimenting with at least some of these to date), the authors have presented a variety of these modifications to better prepare readers for any such changes when they sit the paper. Examples of these modifications include varying the number of options and stems, giving a variety of lead-in instructions and having differing requirements for the number of options required to answer stems. This variety of formats should stress **the importance of carefully reading the entire question** in the examination in case the College employs these variations on a theme again.

The EMIs in this book have been organised into chapters covering the four main subject areas for Part I: psychology and human development, psychopharmacology, descriptive and psychodynamic psychopathology, and clinical theory and skills. Questions within chapters are presented in ascending order of difficulty. This has been done to allow candidates to become familiarised with the EMI format initially with relatively straightforward questions. Once this has been achieved, candidates will be in a position to proceed through the more challenging questions in order to experience some of the more difficult modifications of the basic EMI format and to test the extent of their examination preparedness. The authors expect that the difficulty of the EMIs on the examination paper will lie somewhere between these two extremes.

Readers may note that a number of topics are over-represented among the questions in this book. This is for two main reasons. First, to highlight some of the more important areas of the curriculum that tend to be examined. Second, for pragmatic reasons: EMIs need a list of options, and not all topics lend themselves easily to this. The authors have therefore presented a number of questions on areas that provide such options lists readily (such as the personality disorders), as these are also likely question setting sources for the College composers.

The EMIs provide more scope than the individual statement questions for the test-wise candidate to pick up clues about the possible answer without necessarily knowing anything about the subject matter. An example is the sample EMI provided by the College on aetiology which gives 'having given birth 6 months previously' as an option: two of the stems involve males in the vignettes, thereby allowing the alert candidate to mentally discard one of the options straight away without having to know anything about the question. Options are meant to be brief when composing an EMI, and verbs are avoided in them as this may provide grammatical hints to the candidate. Most of the EMIs in this book are written to avoid these flaws, but some are deliberately designed to incorporate such features. This is to encourage readers to develop test-wise skills, and especially to develop their skill in reading the entire question so as to be able to spot these. Most of the questions set by the College will be of a high standard and will avoid such flaws, but it is inevitable that some will occur, especially as the format is new to both examiners and examinees. You need to be able to pounce upon such cues, as you can be sure many of your colleagues will.

Readers will notice two differences from the College format in a number of EMIs. First, the College presents its options list in a single column, while a number of EMIs in this book lists the options in two columns: this was done both for reasons of space and to provide further variety to challenge the candidate. The authors see it as important that readers are not presented with a standard format of questions in this book, as there will be differences with the actual EMIs encountered in the real examination, and candidates need to be able to adjust to this variety of formats readily. Second, the College has been using three stems per EMI in the examination, while most EMIs in this book have four stems. This was done to provide readers with a sufficient number and variety of questions to prepare for the paper.

To assist candidates in using the EMIs to access textbooks to check material with which they find themselves unfamiliar, the authors have provided a list of the main texts employed as references in preparing these questions. Without exception, the authors recommend all of the texts unreservedly to those studying for the MRCPsych. While it may not be essential for all candidates to have all of these books, a study group ought to have access to most of them, personally or in their training scheme library. With each set of answers to the EMIs, a reference is given, such as: **[G. p136]**, which directs the reader to page 136 of the text listed as 'G' in the reference list. The authors encourage readers to consult these and other texts to refresh areas of unfamiliarity or to check answers that appear incorrect. Note, however, that it is a rare question in psychiatry for which one can only find complete agreement in the literature about its answer.

It is hoped that this work will help fill a gap in trainees' preparations for the MRCPsych Part I written paper. The scarcity of material on EMIs of psychiatry will continue to pose a difficulty for candidates for the immediate future. Various MRCPsych preparation courses will obviously provide material, but this should be supplemented by getting your study group to write EMIs for each other on a regular basis: the questions in this book should give you an idea of how to construct them. Apart from providing extra questions to practise, this exercise will also give you an insight into how EMIs are constructed which can lead to further ideas on how best to answer them. The combination of understanding fully the intricacies of the EMIs, together with knowing your own areas of weakness and directing your study towards remedying these, will mean you should have no fear of the result, as noted above by Sun-Tzu. The authors hope this work will aid you in these goals.

Co. Galway, 2004   M. R.
                                                                            B. R.

References

1. Case SM, Swanson DB. *Constructing Written Test Questions for the Basic and Clinical Sciences,* 3rd edn. Philadelphia: National Board of Medical Examiners, 2001.
2. Sanju G. *Extended Matching Items (EMIs): Solving the Conundrum.* Psychiatric Bulletin 2003; 27: 230–2.
3 http://www.rcpsych.ac.uk/traindev/exams/regulation/emisamp.htm [accessed 5 November 2003]

Acknowledgements

While it is probably foolish to try to thank all who have assisted us with the preparation of this book in some shape or form, since we will undoubtedly forget and offend many, we cannot let the opportunity pass to express our appreciation to the following:

- Our colleagues and other staff in our workplaces, for the numerous examples of support they have given us over the years. In particular we wish to thank our colleagues in the Western Health Board, the Cavan–Monaghan Mental Health Services, the Mid-Western Health Board, the Northern Area Health Board and the INSURE Collaborative Research Project on Suicidal Behaviour.
- Our wives, Samantha and Prabha, for their unfailing understanding and support.
- To our extended families, wherever they may be.
- To Ms. Jennifer Fox for her assistance with the referencing and indexing.

Instructions for Readers

Part of the difficulty of EMIs is that, for a given question, or 'stem', there is often more than one item that is an appropriate 'fit'. Your job is **to select the item that best answers the question**. When you feel you have found an answer to a stem, read through the item list again to ensure there isn't a better one.

One of the authors' aims has been to give a variety of formats of EMI to the reader. EMIs can come in a number of guises and the College is likely to experiment with these until it becomes more familiar with how candidates perform with them. The differing formats in this book are designed so that the reader does not become used to any one style of EMI and to reinforce the absolutely crucial need **to read the entire question exceptionally carefully, in particular the instructions on answering**.

Assume one answer is required per stem unless instructed otherwise: a few of the formats in this book instruct the reader to select two or more answers.

The EMIs in this book are arranged in four chapters to follow the College curriculum for Part I. Within each chapter, **the EMIs are ordered roughly in increasing difficulty**. This is done to allow readers to orient themselves comfortably with the format initially and then to start challenging the boundaries of their knowledge later on. The actual difficulty of the College EMIs is likely to lie between these two extremes.

Each question has a correspondingly numbered answer, explanation and reference at the back of the book. The reference list is a relatively short list of some the most commonly available texts for studying for the MRCPsych Part I. The authors encourage readers strongly **to check any areas of uncertainty in the quoted reference**: in this way they may learn not only what is the right answer, but also why they may have been uncertain.

Psychology and Human Development EMIs

Question 1. Operant conditioning

Theme: Operant conditioning.

Options: A.   After a fixed number of responses.
B.   At random intervals.
C.   At regular intervals.
D.   Constant rate of response.
E.   Fixed ratio schedule.
F.   Rapid rate of response.
G.   Rate of responding has dropped after reinforcement.
H.   Variable interval schedule.
I.   Variable ratio schedule.

Each option may be used once, more than once or not at all.

Lead-in: A 50-year-old woman has played LOTTO every Wednesday and Saturday for the last 30 years with the hope of winning the jackpot. She has won a small amount of money on five occasions in these 30 years. For each of the following choose the concept of operant conditioning above that most closely describes the situation.

Stems: 1.1   The interval at which the reinforcement occurs.

1.2   The main characteristic of her response rate.

1.3   The reinforcement schedule that her behaviour exemplifies.

Question 2. Jean Piaget

Theme: Jean Piaget.

Options: A.   Concrete operations stage.
               B.   Formal operations stage
               C.   Preoperational stage.
               D.   Sensorimotor stage.

Each option may be used once, more than once or not at all.

Lead-in: Choose Piaget's stage of cognitive development above in
               which a child typically develops the characteristic
               behaviours below.

Stems: 2.1   A child develops the concept of time during this stage
                     of Piaget.

               2.2   The game of pretending behaviour in a   child
                     characteristically becomes evident in this stage.

               2.3   The capacity to form mental images develops in this
                     stage.

               2.4   A child's ability to follow multiple displacements of
                     an object, even if the object is hidden within another
                     object, develops in this stage.

Question 3. Concepts of motivation

Theme: Concepts of motivation.

Options: A.   Attitude-discrepant behaviour.
               B.   Cognitive dissonance.
               C.   Drive-reduction theory.
               D.   Glucostatic theory.
               E.   Hierarchy of needs.
               F.   Homeostatic-drive theory.
               G.   Need for achievement.
               H.   Optimal arousal.

Each option may be used once, more than once or not at all.

Lead-in: Each of the following depicts a concept of motivation in humans. Choose the term above for each that most closely fits what is being described.

Stems: 3.1   A senior house officer (SHO) feels he can only study for the MRCPsych examinations in the last few weeks before the papers. He finds that he needs the feeling of time pressure to be able to study efficiently.

               3.2   An SHO wants to become the best psychiatrist she possibly can. She has to put this ambition on hold for the moment, however, as she is on emergency tax since joining a new health trust and she has to find money for food and rent.

               3.3   A specialist registrar (SpR) in psychiatry is notable for her conscientiousness in work. When questioned about this, she reflects and states that she works hard because she enjoys greatly the sense of mastery this diligence brings.

               3.4   An SHO feels he is an excellent psychiatrist but has failed the written paper of Part I on ten occasions. He is strongly motivated to believe that the MRCPsych examinations test only trivia and do not give a fair indication of who is actually a good clinician.

Question 4. Aggression

Theme: Aggression.

Options: A.   Appeasement rituals.
               B.   Catharsis.
               C.   Empathy.
               D.   Incomplete response technique.
               E.   Masochism.
               F.   Modelling.
               G.   Sadism.
               H.   Substitution.
               I.   Sympathy.
               J.   Time-out technique.

Each option may be used once, more than once or not at all.

Lead-in: Crime figures show that violent crimes are more common
               now than they were a few years ago. A number of solutions
               have been suggested to reduce aggression. Choose the
               concept of aggression above that most closely answers each
               of the following.

Stems: 4.1   Practising aggression in harmless ways like playing
                     sports will reduce the violence. This is based on which
                     concept?

               4.2   A child has been sent to his room to prevent his
                     continuing aggressive behaviour. Which technique is
                     being employed?

               4.3   In the Milgram study, when adults were giving
                     electric shocks they were less aggressive when they
                     heard expressions of pain from the victim than when
                     the victim did not make any response. By which
                     concept is this behaviour is explained?

               4.4   Surrendering to prevent aggression in others is an
                     example of which concept?

Question 5. Perception

Theme: Perception.

Options: A.   Adaptation.
                B.   Brain development.
                C.   Four months.
                D.   Habituation.
                E.   Individual learning.
                F.   Nine months.
                G.   Shape constancy.
                H.   Six months.
                I.   Size constancy.

Each option may be used once, more than once or not at all.

Lead-in: Select the option relating to perceptual development and
                constancy above that most closely answers the following.

Stems: 5.1   The ability to see three-dimensional space and to
                      accurately judge distances emerges at about this age
                      in an infant.

                5.2   The nearly universal emergence of depth perception
                      suggests that it is more related to this factor.

                5.3   In the *Ames room* experiment people see the person
                      'shrink' and 'grow' because of this factor.

                5.4   When a stimulus is repeated without change, the
                      orientation response decreases. This response is known
                      as what?

Question 6. *Operant conditioning principles*

Theme: Operant conditioning principles.

Options: A.   Aversive conditioning.
                 B.   Continuous reinforcement.
                 C.   Covert sensitisation.
                 D.   Discrimination.
                 E.   Escape conditioning.
                 F.   Fixed interval reinforcement.
                 G.   Fixed ratio reinforcement.
                 H.   Trial-and-error learning.
                 I.   Variable interval reinforcement.
                 J.   Variable ratio reinforcement.

Each option may be used once only.

Lead-in: For each of the following depictions, select the operant
                 conditioning term above that most closely describes what is
                 occurring.

Stems: 6.1   A senior house officer in psychiatry has no interest in
                       his work, doing the minimum amount of work
                       permissible. He continues in his job because he
                       wants the pay cheque he receives every fortnight.

                 6.2   A man with a recurrent desire for exposing himself
                       in public places manages to keep this impulse under
                       control by frequently imagining vividly that he will
                       be arrested, publicly shamed and put into prison
                       with inmates who attack sex offenders, should he act
                       on his desires.

                 6.3   A woman with alcohol dependence is given a test
                       dose of alcohol after being commenced on disulfiram,
                       since her doctors feel she will not heed their verbal
                       warnings alone.

                 6.4   An assistant bank manager spends much of his spare
                       time fishing. While he agrees the waiting can be
                       boring, he feels the excitement caused by landing a
                       big fish makes it worthwhile.

Question 7. Lobar functions

Theme: Lobar functions.

Options:
    A.   Bilateral parietal lobe lesions.
    B.   Bilateral temporal lobe lesions.
    C.   Frontal and parietal lobe lesions.
    D.   Frontal lesions.
    E.   Left parietal lobe lesions.
    F.   Left temporal lobe lesions.
    G.   Occipital lobe lesions.
    H.   Parieto-occipital lobe lesions.
    I.   Right parietal lobe lesions.
    J.   Right temporal lobe lesions.

Each option may be used once, more than once or not at all.

Lead-in: An 18-year-old girl sustained head injuries in a road traffic accident. She has developed lobar lesions as a result. Choose the lobar involvement above that is/are most likely to be responsible for her symptoms.

Stems:

7.1   She lost her interest in her studies. She started dating numerous men. She is elated but her emotional response is blunted. Her central nervous system examination has revealed a grasp reflex.

7.2   She does not recognise her close relatives' and friends' faces any more. She has right/left disorientation. She finds it difficult to set a table for dinner. She finds it very difficult to do simple calculations. She has astereognosis in both hands.

Question 8. Developmental and hereditary disorders

Theme: Developmental and hereditary disorders with neuropsychiatric manifestations.

Options: A. Acute intermittent porphyria.
B. Adrenoleukodystrophy.
C. Down's syndrome.
D. Fragile X syndrome.
E. Huntington's disease.
F. Learning disorder of the right hemisphere.
G. Metachromatic leukodystrophy.
H. Olivopontocerebellar degeneration.
I. Prader-Willi syndrome.

Each option may be used once, more than once or not at all.

Lead-in: For each of the neuropsychiatric syndromes described below, select the disorder above that is most likely to be responsible for the findings.

Stems: 8.1 X-linked female heterozygotes may manifest mild learning disability, hyperactivity, affective disorder, and developmental Gerstmann syndrome.

8.2 This autosomal dominant chromosomal disease typically occurs in middle age and is characterised by movement disorder and subcortical dementia. Sufferers are prone to develop mood disorders.

8.3 This autosomal dominant disease occurs usually in the third decade and is characterised by intermittent attacks of abdominal pain, polyneuropathy, seizures and delirium.

8.4 This hereditary chromosomal disease is the second most common cause of learning disability in men. The male has a characteristic face and may develop autism. Learning disability becomes obvious when the child begins school.

Question 9. Concepts of aggression

Theme: Concepts of aggression.

Options: A.   Aggressive cue theory.   F.   Hostile aggression.
                B.   Appeasement gestures.   G.   Instrumental aggression.
                C.   Deindividuation.   H.   Ritualisation.
                D.   Fighting instinct.   I.   Social learning theory.
                E.   Frustration-aggression   J.   Thanatos.
                     hypothesis.

Each option may be used once, more than once or not at all.

Lead-in: For each of the following scenarios depicting a concept of
                theories of aggression, select the term above which most
                closely describes the concept.

Stems: 9.1   Each individual has an innate death instinct. This is
                      initially directed towards the individual himself, but
                      later in life it is displaced towards others and can thus
                      result in overt aggression.

                9.2   Humans have some actions, such as bowing to a
                      leader, which are thought to mirror the actions of
                      some animals whereby aggressive events are avoided.

                9.3   When an individual is thwarted in his desires, this
                      leads to negative feelings. As such negative feelings
                      build up, it becomes inevitable that this will
                      eventually lead to aggressive behaviour.

                9.4   A large-scale riot occurs at a soccer match. At the
                      trials arising out of this, it is noticeable that there
                      were many individuals who rioted who had no
                      previous history of aggression and who were described
                      as normally placid by those who knew them.

Question 10. *Concepts of classical and operant conditioning*

Theme: Concepts of classical and operant conditioning.

Options: A.   Continuous reinforcement.
                B.   Chaining.
                C.   Discrimination.
                D.   Extinction.
                E.   Forward conditioning.
                F.   Habituation.
                G.   Incubation.
                H.   Preparedness.
                I.   Shaping.
                J.   Simultaneous conditioning.
                K.   Stimulus generalisation.
                L.   Trace conditioning.

Each option may be used once only.

Lead-in: For each of the following descriptions, select the term
                above that it most closely exemplifies.

Stems: 10.1   A parent wishes to teach a child to put his toys away
                        into his toy chest. The child is rewarded successively
                        over time for putting his toys away into his room,
                        then for putting them into the cupboard, then for
                        putting them into the toy chest in the cupboard.

                10.2   A rat has learned to push a lever to receive food
                        when a light shines. Food has stopped coming
                        recently, however, and the rat no longer pushes the
                        lever.

                10.3   A light is switched on briefly then extinguished
                        before a cat is given an electric shock five seconds
                        later. Over a period of time the cat learns to have a
                        fear response to the subsequent appearances of the
                        light.

                10.4   An experimenter tries to develop a treatment for
                        nicotine addiction by attempting to create a phobia
                        for cigarettes but finds it much more difficult than if
                        one were trying to create a phobia for mice.

Question 11. Concepts associated with Piaget

Theme: Concepts associated with Piaget.

Options:

A.	Accommodation.	G.	Laws of conservation.
B.	Animism.	H.	Object permanence.
C.	Artificialism.	I.	Precausal reasoning.
D.	Assimilation.	J.	Propositional thought.
E.	Circular reactions.	K.	Schema.
F.	Egocentrism.	L.	Syncretism.

Each option may be used once, more than once or not at all.

Lead-in: For each of the following children, select the term above that best describes the concept from Piaget's theories being demonstrated.

Stems:

11.1 A four-year-old girl cries when she sees that her father has bumped his car against the wall because 'the car is hurt!'

11.2 A three-year-old boy has a box on his head. He is pleased with this hiding place as he assumes that, since he can't see others, they cannot see him.

11.3 A nine-month-old girl has recently begun to look over the side of her highchair to where she has just thrown her rattle.

11.4 An eight-year-old boy realises that when liquid is poured from a wide, short beaker into a narrow, tall one, the volume of liquid in both is the same.

Question 12. Agnosias

Theme: Agnosias.

Options: A.   Agraphognosia.   F.   Colour agnosia.
               B.   Anosodiaphoria.   G.   Finger agnosia.
               C.   Anosognosia.   H.   Hemisomatognosia.
               D.   Astereognosia.   I.   Prosopagnosia.
               E.   Autotopagnosia.   J.   Simultanagnosia.

Each option may be used once, more than once or not at all.

Lead-in: For each of the following vignettes select the required
               number of agnosias above that are being displayed.

Stems: 12.1   A young man looks at a picture and can tell that
                      various elements are of different colours but cannot
                      name these colours. He can also point out that there
                      are mountains and people in the picture but does not
                      realise that a scene of mountain climbing is being
                      depicted. (Two items)

               12.2   An elderly woman looks into a mirror and cannot
                      recognise who is looking back at her. (One item)

               12.3   A middle-aged man is asked to point to various body
                      parts such as his foot, knee and ear by the clinician,
                      but is unable to comply with these instructions. (One
                      item)

               12.4   An elderly woman has developed recently a marked
                      hemiplegia. She is aware of the change in her
                      mobility and what has caused it but is completely
                      unconcerned about it. (One item)

Question 13. Moral development

Theme: Moral development.

Options:
    A.   Autonomous morality.
    B.   Conventional morality.
    C.   Heteronomous morality.
    D.   Induction.
    E.   Love withdrawal.
    F.   Morality of care.
    G.   Morality of justice.
    H.   Post-conventional morality.
    I.   Power assertion.
    J.   Pre-conventional morality.
    K.   Pre-moral period.

Each option may be used once, more than once or not at all.

Lead-in: Choose the concept of the development of morality that best fits each of the following statements.

Stems:

13.1   In Piaget's cognitive developmental theory of moral development, a child believes in reciprocal punishment at this stage.

13.2   In Kohlberg's cognitive development theory, a child believes in obeying the rules of those in authority at this stage of moral development.

13.3   Gilligan proposed that boys develop this type of morality.

13.4   This is a very ineffective parenting style for promoting the moral development of children.

Question 14. *Theories of language development*

Theme: Theories of language development.

Options: A.   Babbling.
               B.   Critical-period.
               C.   Holophrastic period.
               D.   Language acquisition device.
               E.   Linguistic universals.
               F.   Motherese.
               G.   Over-extension.
               H.   Over-regularisation.
               I.   Pragmatics.
               J.   Prelinguistic stage.
               K.   Telegraphic period.
               L.   Transformational grammar.

Each option may be used once, more than once or not at all.

Lead-in: For each of the following depictions of a concept of
               language development, choose the term above that most
               closely fits the description.

Stems: 14.1   A 20-month-old girl reacts angrily to a visitor who
                      unwittingly uses the child's father's favourite cup
                      for tea. The girl points and shouts repeatedly:
                      "Daddy cup".

               14.2   An 11-month-old girl lying in her cot while playing
                      with a soft toy constantly repeats: "da-da-da-da-da-
                      da".

               14.3   On a walk, a woman points out a cow and teaches
                      her 15-month-old son to say this word. The next day
                      he spots a horse and, pointing, shouts excitedly:
                      "cow!"

               14.4   Two Finnish-speaking children are orphaned and are
                      sent to live with an aunt and uncle who live in
                      Scotland. The 5-year-old boy has little difficulty in
                      learning flawless English (with a noticeable Scottish
                      accent) in comparison to his 14-year-old brother.

Question 15. Interpersonal attractiveness

Theme: Interpersonal attractiveness.

Options: A.   Both genders.
B.   Competence.
C.   Female.
D.   High disclosure.
E.   High self-monitors.
F.   Low self-monitors.
G.   Male.
H.   Moderate disclosure.
I.   Physical attractiveness.
J.   Similarity.

Each option may be used once, more than once or not at all.

Lead-in: Choose the term above from psychological theories of what makes an individual socially popular and successful that best answers each of the following statements.

Stems: 15.1   Physical attractiveness has more influence on the fate of this gender(s) in dating.

15.2   This is the main factor that determines friendship.

15.3   This amount of self-disclosure leads to reciprocity.

15.4   With this level of self-monitoring, individuals try to accurately present their beliefs and principles no matter what the situation is.

Question 16. *Problem-solving and decision-making*

Theme: Problem-solving and decision-making.

Options: A.   Availability heuristic.
B.   Convergent thinking.
C.   Divergent thinking.
D.   Lateral thinking.
E.   Negative transfer effect.
F.   Positive transfer effect.
G.   Representativeness bias.
H.   Trial-and-error learning.

Each option may be used once, more than once or not at all.

Lead-in: Each of the following represents a concept of problem-solving or decision-making. Select the term above that best describes the concept being depicted.

Stems: 16.1   Some children are playing a game in school. One boy is asked a series of questions, the answer to all of which is 'silk'. When he is then asked what cows drink, he answers confidently: 'milk!'

16.2   A lever in a cage releases some food when pressed. A rat eventually discovers this and thereafter presses the lever whenever she is hungry.

16.3   A class of 15-year-old teenagers is asked how likely it is that tourists to Israel would be attacked by terrorists. Most significantly overestimate the risk.

16.4   A female experimenter is in a locked room with a male subject who is given a pole, some wire, a rope and a dishcloth. She explains to him the object of the test is to use the materials to escape from the room to win a reward of £100. She is somewhat taken aback when he picks up the pole and threatens to hit her over the head unless she releases him. Having got out, he calmly asks her for his prize.

Question 17. Learning theory

Theme: Learning theory.

Options: A. Aversion.
B. Covert sensitisation.
C. Extinction.
D. Flooding.
E. Mowrer's two-factor theory.
F. Pavlov's classical conditioning.
G. Primary reinforcer.
H. Reciprocal inhibition.
I. Secondary reinforcer.
J. Skinner's operant conditioning.

Each option may be used once, more than once or not at all.

Lead-in: Which of the terms above best describe the concepts of learning theory set out below?

Stems: 17.1 Cue exposure for the treatment of drug abuse is based on this principle.

17.2 The techniques of exposure and response prevention are based on this theory.

17.3 Food, when it is used as a reinforcer, is defined as this type of reinforcer.

17.4 The technique of reducing anxiety provided by imagining the phobic situation coupled with relaxation is an example of this behavioural therapy.

Question 18. Gender development

Theme: Gender development.

Options: A.   Androgyny.   F.   Gender schemas.
              B.   Basic gender identity. G.   Gender stability.
              C.   Electra complex.   H.   Oedipus complex.
              D.   Gender consistency.   I.   Sex role.
              E.   Gender identity.   J.   Sexual identity.

Each option may be used once only.

Lead-in: For each of the following descriptions of a concept of
              gender development, select the term above that most
              closely describes the depiction.

Stems: 18.1   Girls discover that they do not have penises around
                     the age of three. They begin to love their fathers
                     more than their mothers and begin to fantasise
                     about having their father's baby.

              18.2   A three-year-old boy knows he is a boy but tells his
                     mother that he will be a beautiful woman just like
                     her when he grows up.

              18.3   The most balanced individuals are those who can
                     utilise either masculine or feminine characteristics
                     as the situation demands, and who do not have to
                     suppress certain characteristics because they do not
                     fit the conventional stereotype.

              18.4   Certain biological factors dictate the gender of the
                     individual, such as the penis and scrotum in the
                     male.

Question 19. Goffman's theories of institutionalisation

Theme: Goffman's theories of institutionalisation.

Options:

A.	Batch living.	F.	Mortification process.
B.	Betrayal funnel.	G.	Patient role.
C.	Binary living.	H.	Role-stripping.
D.	Institutional perspective.	I.	Total institution.
E.	Moral career.		

Each option may be used once, more than once or not at all.

Lead-in: For each of the following vignettes, select the term from Goffman above that it most closely depicts.

Stems:

19.1 The family of a 55-year-old man consult with his family doctor of many years to initiate having him committed involuntarily to a psychiatric institution.

19.2 The man arrives for admission to the psychiatric institution. The nurses ask him to give up his belongings so that they can be itemised and put away. They then ask him to get into pyjamas so that the doctor can examine him.

19.3 One of his resentments over the following months is that he can see staff enjoying tea and cigarettes whenever they like and that they get to go home daily, while the patients have to stay put and only get such treats at allotted times.

19.4 Over the years, his self-esteem gradually suffers and he sees himself and the other patients as inferior to the institution staff.

Question 20. Visual perception

Theme: Visual perception.

Options: A.   Binocular vision.
B.   Colour constancy.
C.   Convergence.
D.   Figure ground differentiation.
E.   Law of closure.
F.   Law of proximity.
G.   Law of similarity.
H.   Linear perspective.
I.   Location constancy.
J.   Motion parallax.
K.   Size constancy.
L.   Shape constancy.

Each option may be used once, more than once or not at all.

Lead-in: For each of the following depictions, select the term above that most closely describes the concept of visual perception being demonstrated.

Stems: 20.1   A child in the back seat of a car travelling north notices that the telephone poles along the side of the road appear to be moving south in contrast to a far-off hill which appears to be going north.

20.2   A child alternates her gaze from looking at a cow in the next field to trying to look at the tip of her own nose.

20.3   A card with a figure is held up to a child for a few seconds. She states that she has seen a complete circle, but on inspecting the card later, she notes that the figure is indeed circular but has a gap in it.

20.4   A child is shown a square piece of card at an angle such that the base is nearest the child and the card slopes backwards to the adult holding it. Despite this, she perceives it to be a square.

Question 21. Behaviour modification

Theme: Behaviour modification.

Options: A.   Exposure in virtual reality.
   B.   Eye movement desensitisation.
   C.   Imaginal flooding.
   D.   Imaginal systematic desensitisation.
   E.   Implosion.
   F.   *In vivo* flooding.
   G.   Interoceptive exposure.
   H.   Response prevention.
   I.   Self-directed exposure.

Each option may be used once, more than once or not at all.

Lead-in: Select the term above that most closely describes the behavioural modification techniques depicted below.

Stems: 21.1   A 40-year-old female with a fear of eating in public was instructed to eat her meal in front of professional people, who were observing her behaviour.

   21.2   The exposure to both imagined and remembered events in order to overcome a fear.

   21.3   A patient with fear of hospitals is treated with a programmed practice hierarchy of situations involving decreasing distances to a hospital, to be completed over time by himself with support from his wife.

Question 22. Concepts of attachment

Theme: Concepts of attachment.

Options: A.   Affectionless psychopathy.
                 B.   Affiliation.
                 C.   Anxious-avoidant attachment.
                 D.   Anxious-resistant attachment.
                 E.   Bonding.
                 F.   Imprinting.
                 G.   Indiscriminate attachment phase.
                 H.   Multiple attachment phase.
                 I.   Pre-attachment phase.
                 J.   Secure attachment.

Each option may be used once, more than once or not at all.

Lead-in: For each of the following scenarios, select the term above
                 from attachment theory that most closely describes what is
                 being depicted.

Stems: 22.1   In the hours and days after birth, a mother stares
                        contentedly at her baby girl in her arms.

                 22.2   In the *Strange Situation* experiment, a baby shows
                        little interest when his mother leaves the room but
                        becomes upset when the stranger also leaves. He can
                        be comforted by both his mother and the stranger
                        when upset.

                 22.3   An ten-week-old baby girl smiles at all the old
                        women in the post office who stick their heads into
                        her pram and make faces at her, just as much as she
                        smiles at her proud parents standing nearby.

                 22.4   A woman who hates going to the dentist asks her
                        friend to accompany her when she has to have an
                        extraction.

Question 23. *Theory of emotion*

Theme: Theory of emotion.

Options: A.   Bodily arousal follows a feeling.
               B.   Bodily arousal is interpreted on the basis of experience and situation cues.
               C.   By attributing bodily arousal to a particular cue.
               D.   Emotional feelings and bodily arousal arise simultaneously from the actions of the thalamus.
               E.   Emotional feelings follow bodily arousal.
               F.   Evaluating personal meanings of a situation results in specific emotions.
               G.   Facial expressions feedback defining the feelings.

Each option may be used once, more than once or not at all.

Lead-in: An athlete who won a gold medal in the Olympics was overjoyed. Tears of happiness rolled down his face. How do emotional feelings occur? How are feelings interrelated to expressions, arousal, behaviour and thoughts?

               The following theories attempt to answer these questions. Choose the statement above that most closely describes the main concept of the theory below.

Stems: 23.1   The James-Lang theory suggests this.

               23.2   The Cannon-Bard theory suggests this.

               23.3   The emotional appraisal theory suggests this.

               23.4   Schachter's cognitive theory suggests this.

Question 24. Personality assessment

Theme: Personality assessment.

Options: A.   Comrey personality scales (CPS).
               B.   Eysenck personality questionnaire (EPQ).
               C.   Figure Drawing Test.
               D.   Holtzman Inkblot Technique (HIT).
               E.   Minnesota Multiphasic Personality Inventory 2
                     (MMPI-2).
               F.   Personality Assessment Inventory (PAI).
               G.   Rorschach Test.
               H.   Sentence Completion Test.
               I.   16 Personality Factor Questionnaire (16 PF).
               J.   Thematic Apperception Test (TAT).

Each option may be used once, more than once or not at all.

Lead-in: Select the personality test above that is being described in
               the following.

Stems: 24.1   This short scale that has theoretical validity is a
                      simple, self-report format, screening device. It has a
                      theoretical basis and research support. Its items are
                      transparent as to purpose.

               24.2   This self-report format with dimensional scales is a
                      sophisticated psychometric instrument with
                      considerable research conduced on non-clinical
                      populations.

               24.3   This projective test involves administering twenty
                      cards depicting a number of scenes of varying
                      ambiguity.

               24.4   This test involves completing written responses to
                      half-written statements. The stimuli are obvious in
                      intent and subject to easy falsification.

Question 25. Prejudice

Theme:　　Prejudice.

Options:　　A.　Authoritarian personality.
　　　　　　　　B.　Contact hypothesis.
　　　　　　　　C.　Egoistic deprivation.
　　　　　　　　D.　Ethnocentrism.
　　　　　　　　E.　Fraternalistic deprivation.
　　　　　　　　F.　Frustration-aggression hypothesis.
　　　　　　　　G.　Realistic conflict theory.
　　　　　　　　H.　Social identity theory.
　　　　　　　　I.　System theory.

Each option may be used once, more than once or not at all.

Lead-in:　　Prejudice is a negative attitude towards the members of some groups based solely on their membership of that group. Choose the concept above that most closely fits the following statements.

Stems:　　25.1　The theory of Adorno and others of prejudice is based on this concept.

　　　　　　　25.2　The most extreme racist attitudes among town dwellers in the United States were found in a study to show the highest levels of this factor.

　　　　　　　25.3　The reduction in prejudice among white and black housewives living close to each other supports this theory.

　　　　　　　25.4　When the members of two groups compete for the same goal, they become prejudiced against each other. This concept is the core principle of this theory.

Question 26. Stages of development

Theme: Stages of development.

Options: A.   Development is at the lower limit of the range of normal development.

B.   Development is at the upper limit of the range of normal development.

C.   Development is earlier than one would expect for the child's age.

D.   Development is later than one would expect for the child's age.

E.   Development is within normal limits.

F.   Insufficient information is given to judge developmental stage.

Each option may be used once, more than once or not at all.

Lead-in: For each of the following children, choose the phrase above that *most closely* describes the stage of development he/she most recently attained.

Stems: 26.1   A thirty-month-old boy has just learned to look down from his highchair when he throws his toys on the ground, to see where they have gone. Prior to this, he ignored them when they fell.

26.2   An excited househusband calls his wife at work to tell her that their seventeen-month-old son has just learned how to take six whole steps unaided.

26.3   An eighteen-month-old girl expresses her displeasure at her empty mug by shouting 'milk gone!' This is the first time she has used two words together.

26.4   A twelve-year-old girl can repeat backwards five numbers that have just been called out to her.

Question 27. Self-concept and growth

Theme: Self-concept and growth.

Options: A. Conditions of worth.
        B. Deficit motivation.
        C. Efficacy expectations.
        D. Growth motivation.
        E. Interpret his personal construct.
        F. Negative regard.
        G. Outcome expectation.
        H. Positive regard.
        I. Reinterpret his personal construct.
        J. Safety needs.

Each option may be used once, more than once or not at all.

Lead-in: The following descriptions of self-belief, need and motivation are based on one of the above-mentioned principles, concepts or mechanisms.

Stems: 27.1 According to Bandura, people who consider more options and pursue their goal successfully have this belief.

          27.2 George Kelly's construct theory proposes that a person can change his behaviour by being helped to undergo this procedure.

          27.3 According to Maslow, satisfying this motivation often results in increased tension.

          27.4 According to Rogers, this is a basic need of all people.

Question 28. *Prosocial behaviour*

Theme: Prosocial behaviour.

Options: A.   Arousal–cost–reward model.
                B.   Biological altruism.
                C.   Diffusion of responsibility.
                D.   Empathy-altruism hypothesis.
                E.   Genuine ambiguity.
                F.   Negative-state relief model.
                G.   Pluralistic ignorance.
                H.   Psychological altruism.
                I.   Reciprocity norm.
                J.   Universal egoism.

Each option may be used once, more than once or not at all.

Lead-in: For each of the following descriptions, choose the concept
                of prosocial behaviour above that most closely represents
                what is being depicted.

Stems: 28.1   Many neighbours on a housing estate see one of their
                       neighbours running in terror from a man who is
                       brandishing a knife, yet only one person rings the
                       police and no one intervenes.

                28.2   A group of students are taking their summer
                       examinations in a large hall when the fire alarm goes
                       off and some smoke appears. Not wishing to be
                       alarmed unnecessarily, a number of students look
                       around to see the reactions of others and, seeing no
                       commotion, continue answering their papers.

                28.3   When one sees another individual in distress and
                       empathises with them, this causes the observer to
                       feel sad as a result. It is an attempt to alleviate this
                       personal sadness that leads the observer to act in an
                       altruistic fashion, rather than empathetic concerns.

                28.4   During an office-block fire many individuals who
                       were working in the building start helping others to
                       escape in an almost reflexive way while placing
                       themselves in considerable danger.

Question 29. Theories of moral development

Theme: Theories of moral development.

Options: A. Approval/disapproval orientation.
B. Authority orientation.
C. Ethical principle orientation.
D. Morality of care.
E. Morality of justice.
F. Moral realism.
G. Moral relativism.
H. Punishment orientation.
I. Reward orientation.
J. Social contract orientation.

Each option may be used once, more than once or not at all.

Lead-in: For each of the following statements, chose the most closely concept of moral development above that it describes.

Stems: 29.1 According to Piaget, a seven-year-old tends to believe that rules must be observed at all costs. Punishment should depend on the severity of the crime and it should always occur when a crime is committed.

29.2 According to Kohlberg, individuals can reach a stage in their moral development in which they tend to act to avoid the disapproval of those in commanding positions and because they wish to fulfil their obligations.

29.3 According to Kohlberg, individuals can reach a stage in their moral development in which they tend to act to avoid disappointing themselves by upholding a series of beliefs about issues such as fairness and equality.

29.4 According to Gilligan, females may be considered artefactually at a lower level of moral development on Kohlberg's stages because they tend to display a consideration for the wellbeing of others.

Question 30. Perception and cognition

Theme: Perception and cognition.

Options: A.   Both conscious and non-conscious perceptions.
                B.   Categorising dimension of selective attention.
                C.   Conscious perceptions only.
                D.   Declarative memory.
                E.   Explicit memory.
                F.   Filtering dimension of selective attention.
                G.   Implicit memory.
                H.   Non-conscious perceptions only.
                I.   Parallel processes.
                J.   Pigeonholing dimension of selective attention.
                K.   Serial processes.

Each option may be used once, more than once or not at all.

Lead-in: Which of the above perceptual and cognitive terms refers
                to the following statements?

Stems: 30.1   Patients with schizophrenia show greater difficulty
                        with this dimension of selective attention when
                        they are symptomatic.

                30.2   Long-term memory can encode these types of
                        perceptions.

                30.3   This type of memory cannot be expressed in words.

                30.4   In processing a stimulus, this type of process has
                        low processing capacity demands.

Question 31. Psychological testing

Theme: Psychological testing.

Options:
A. Clock Drawing.
B. Digit Span.
C. Finger Tapping.
D. MMPI.*
E. National Adult Reading Test.
F. Rey-Osterrieth Complex Figure.
G. Rorschach.
H. Stroop Test.
I. Thematic Apperception Test.
J. Trail-Making Test.

Each option may be used once, more than once or not at all.

Lead-in: A 65-year-old man with altered behaviour over the last eight months is referred for psychological assessment. Choose the appropriate tests above to answer the following questions.

Stems: 31.1 The psychologist has been asked to perform projective personality testing on the patient.

Which tests could he perform for this?

31.2 Before he starts, however, the psychologist wants to get a quick indication of the patient's attention and concentration to gauge how well he will engage with the assessment.

Which test could he perform for this?

31.3 The psychologist wishes to get an estimate of the patient's premorbid intelligence quotient.

Which test could he perform for this?

31.4 The patient's family have noticed him to be apathetic yet impulsive over the last eight months. He tends to be irritable and uses coarse language frequently, which is very unusual for him. His judgement tends to be poor and they have noticed him make tactless remarks to complete strangers on occasion.

Which tests is the psychologist most likely to carry out in light of this collateral information?

*Minnesota Multiphasic Personality Inventory.

Question 32. Behaviour theory

Theme: Behaviour theory.

Options:
A. Aversion theory.
B. Classical conditioning.
C. False.
D. Modelling principle.
E. Instrumental conditioning.
F. Premack principle.
G. Sitting in the chair.
H. Social interaction.
I. Social learning theory.
J. True.

Each option may be used once, more than once or not at all.

Lead-in: A 40-year-old woman in a psychiatric hospital spent all her waking hours sitting in one particular chair. She rarely interacted with other people. The hospital staff shaped her behaviour to spend more time in social interactions by permitting her to sit in her favourite chair only after spending a specified amount of time with others.

Using the above terms, answer the following questions as to how behaviour theory relates to this scenario.

Stems:

32.1 Which principle has this reinforcing procedure followed?

32.2 Based on that principle, which is the high-probability behaviour that the woman performs?

32.3 The intervention selected is based on which concept of learning theory?

32.4 Is it correct that in order for the high-probability behaviour to reinforce the low-probability behaviour, the high-frequency behaviour must be pleasurable?

Question 33. Behaviour therapy

Theme: Behaviour therapy.

Options: A.   Conditional reinforcer.
B.   Contextual stimuli.
C.   Contrived reinforcer.
D.   Counterconditioning.
E.   Extinction.
F.   Latent inhibition.
G.   Natural reinforcer.
H.   Postconditioning revaluation of the unconditioned stimulus.
I.   Second-order conditioning.

Each option may be used once, more than once or not at all.

Lead-in: The following behaviour interventions are based on which of the above mechanisms?

Stems: 33.1   Overcoming a spider phobia with treatment, associated with diminishing the fear of places where spiders reside, involves this mechanism.

33.2   A public recital of a piece of music that reinforces further artistic behaviour in the individual is an example of this type of reinforcer.

33.3   A child fears cats. The pairing of his being confronted with a cat at the same time as being given some sweets is an example of this concept.

33.4   Pre-exposure of patients with cancer to the chemotherapy environment to reduce the later aversive response to the environment involves this principle.

Question 34. Concepts of forgetting

Theme: Concepts of forgetting.

Options: A.   Context-dependent forgetting.
                 B.   Cue-dependent forgetting.
                 C.   Decay theory.
                 D.   Displacement theory.
                 E.   Interference theory.
                 F.   Motivated interference.
                 G.   Proactive inhibition.
                 H.   Retrieval failure.
                 I.   Retroactive inhibition.
                 J.   State-dependent forgetting.
                 K.   Storage failure.
                 L.   Trace-strength diminishment.

Each option may be used once only or not at all.

Lead-in: For each of the following descriptions of forgetting, select
                 the theory or process above that most closely describes the
                 phenomenon.

Stems: 34.1   A 12-year-old boy can recite his poetry homework
                        perfectly when in his room with his stereo playing,
                        but recalls only bits of it when asked to recite it
                        elsewhere.

                 34.2   A 24-year-old woman finds it difficult to remember
                        large portions of her childhood but notes that she
                        had suffered recurrent violent abuse from her
                        father.

                 34.3   A 37-year-old man has moved recently from
                        Scotland to the United States. When driving to work,
                        he frequently finds himself getting into the
                        passenger side of the car.

                 34.4   A 71-year-old man hears a noise downstairs and fears
                        there is an intruder. He suddenly remembers long-
                        forgotten aspects of being attacked in his house years
                        earlier.

Question 35. Behavioural analysis

Theme: Behavioural analysis.

Options:
    A.   Classical conditioning.
    B.   Consequent operation.
    C.   Establishing operation.
    D.   Instrumental conditioning.
    E.   Learned helplessness.
    F.   Operant conditioning.
    G.   Orienting response.
    H.   Shaping.
    I.   Signalling operation.
    J.   Stimulus presentation operation.

Each option may be used once, more than once or not at all.

Lead-in: A dog is conditioned to salivate when the sound from a bell is presented before some food.

Answer the following questions using the terms from learning theory above.

Stems:
    35.1   Which term refers to the dog's response for the first time to the sound from the bell before the food is presented?

    35.2   Which type of operation is the presentation of the conditional stimulus?

    35.3   Which type of operation is the presentation of the unconditional stimulus?

    35.4   Of which type of conditioning is the procedure described above an example?

Question 36. Theories and concepts of emotion

Theme: Theories and concepts of emotion.

Options: A.   Affective primacy theory.
              B.   Cannon-Bard theory.
              C.   Cognitive appraisal theory.
              D.   Cognitive labelling theory.
              E.   Facial feedback hypothesis.
              F.   False feedback paradigm.
              G.   Feeling rules.
              H.   James-Lange theory.
              I.   Misattribution effect.
              J.   Neural hijack.

Each option may be used once, more than once or not at all.

Lead-in: For each of the following accounts, select the
              theory/concept of emotion above it describes most closely.

Stems: 36.1   A man crosses a road without looking and has to run
                      out of the way quickly when the driver of a lorry
                      sounds his horn angrily at him. Because of this
                      activity of running away, the man experiences the
                      emotion of fear.

              36.2   A tourist is walking down a street in Belfast when a
                      child bursts a balloon behind him. The man
                      experiences terror because his first thought was that
                      a bomb had exploded.

              36.3   A woman agrees to take part in an experiment. She
                      agrees to smile at every second photograph she is
                      shown. When she is asked to recall which of the
                      scenes were happy ones, she tends to mention the
                      scenes she 'smiled' at.

              36.4   For fear responses, the amygdala sends impulses to
                      most areas of the brain such as the motor cortex and
                      the brain stem, thereby ensuring the coordination of
                      the physical and emotional responses to a fearful
                      stimulus.

Question 37. Neurodevelopment

Theme: Neurodevelopment.

Options: A.   Drawing test.
               B.   Gross motor skill levels.
               C.   Intellectual quotient.
               D.   Language development.
               E.   Motor development.
               F.   Motor quotient.
               G.   Sensory quotient.
               H.   Social milestones.
               I.   Visual milestones.
               J.   Weschler Intelligence Scale for Children – III.

Each option may be used once, more than once or not at all.

Lead-in: Which of the above developmental events, psychological tests or test findings best fit the following statements?

Stems: 37.1   In the absence of a communication disorder or significant hearing impairment this is the best predictor of future intellectual development.

               37.2   This is an easy, non-threatening test for school-going children to assess their graphomotor abilities.

               37.3   The cut-off point for serious disability is lower for this development than for other streams of development.

               37.4   This is the functional expression of the cumulative impact of language comprehension and problem-solving skills.

Question 38. Social influence

Theme: Social influence.

Options: A.   Audience effect.
              B.   Autocratic leadership.
              C.   Coercive social power.
              D.   Democratic leadership.
              E.   Diffusion of responsibility.
              F.   Expert social power.
              G.   Groupthink.
              H.   Informational social influence.
              I.   Normative social influence.
              J.   Pluralistic ignorance.
              K.   Referent social power.
              L.   Task-oriented leadership.

Each option may be used once, more than once or not at all.

Lead-in: For each of the following scenarios, choose the term above that best describes the concept of social influence being demonstrated.

Stems: 38.1 The managing director of a paper supply firm tends to be domineering in his relations with staff. He is more interested in getting the job done than his interpersonal relationships with staff. When questioned about whom he likes least to work with, he strongly criticises his assistant managing director.

              38.2 A community mental health team calls a meeting to review its policies after ten suicides of patients in two months. Despite many misgivings being expressed early in the meeting about practices, members of the group as a whole convince each other that there are no problems to be concerned about and no one is really to blame.

              38.3 A consultant psychiatrist is very highly regarded in her health authority as she has by far the best knowledge of the Mental Health Act. Others tend to turn to her for advice when legal grey areas arise.

              38.4 A senior house officer tends to perform a much better examination of the central nervous system when observed by his consultant than when he is doing it alone in casualty.

Psychopharmacology EMIs

Question 39. *Physical emergencies during antipsychotic treatment*

Theme: Physical emergencies during antipsychotic treatment.

Options: A.   Change his antipsychotic to a different group.
B.   Creatinine phosphokinase (CPK).
C.   Discontinue his antipsychotic.
D.   Fifty per cent.
E.   Increase his antipsychotic drug dose.
F.   Liver function tests (LFTs).
G.   Neuroleptic malignant syndrome.
H.   Oneiroid state.
I.   Renal function tests (RFTs).
J.   Septicaemia.
K.   Ten per cent.
L.   Thirty per cent.

Each option may be used once, more than once or not at all.

Lead-in: A 40-year-old man who has been on a typical antipsychotic for the last ten days has developed motor rigidity, fever, sweating, agitation and disorientation.

Using the above terms, answer the following questions about this emergency situation.

Stems: 39.1   What is the most likely reason for this clinical picture?

39.2   Which blood test would you order to confirm your diagnosis?

39.3   If your diagnosis were confirmed, what would be your immediate step in altering his prescription?

39.4   What is the mortality rate of this condition?

Question 40. Extrapyramidal side-effects

Theme: Extrapyramidal side-effects.

Options: A.   After three months.
                 B.   After two weeks.
                 C.   Akathisia.
                 D.   Bradykinesia.
                 E.   Dystonia.
                 F.   Elevated creatinine phosphokinase levels.
                 G.   Hyperbilirubinaemia.
                 H.   Parkinsonism.
                 I.   Reticulocytosis.
                 J.   Rigidity.
                 K.   Tremor.
                 L.   Within five days.

Each option may be used once, more than once or not at all.

Lead-in: A 25-year-old male has a two-year history of hearing
                 voices commenting on his behaviour, and persecutory
                 ideas that aliens are trying to abduct him. He was noted to
                 be smiling inappropriately and was unkempt. He was
                 commenced on haloperidol.

                 *Using the above, select the term that most closely answers the
                 following questions about extrapyramidal side-effects.*

Stems: 40.1   He developed torticollis of his neck, an occulogyric
                        crisis and mild opisthotonus. What was the most
                        likely time frame for him to develop these
                        symptoms?

                 40.2   Which extrapyramidal effect always responds to
                        treatment with an anticholinergic?

                 40.3   Symptoms of severe rigidity, increased
                        temperature, confusion and autonomic instability
                        are associated with which haematological findings?

                 40.4   In drug-induced Parkinsonism, which clinical sign
                        predominates?

Question 41. Antipsychotics

Theme: Antipsychotics.

Options: A.   Clozapine.
              B.   Droperidol.
              C.   Flupenthixol.
              D.   Olanzapine.
              E.   Pimozide.
              F.   Quetiapine.
              G.   Risperidone.
              H.   Sulpiride.
              I.   Trifluoperazine.
              J.   Ziprasidone.

Each option may be used once, more than once or not at all.

Lead-in: For each of the following statements about adverse effects
              of antipsychotics, choose the drug above that is most
              likely to be implicated.

Stems: 41.1   A common side-effect of this thienobenzodiazepine
                     atypical antipsychotic is weight gain.

              41.2   This dibenzothiazepine atypical antipsychotic is not
                     associated with any significant increase in serum
                     prolactin levels.

              41.3   This substituted benzamide antipsychotic is
                     thought to have a dose-dependant action at
                     presynaptic dopamine sites.

              41.4   This diphenylbutylpiperidine is the longest-acting
                     per oral administered antipsychotic.

Question 42. Pharmacokinetics

Theme: Pharmacokinetics.

Options: A.   Extraction ratio for a drug by a specific organ.
              B.   First-order kinetics.
              C.   Total clearance.
              D.   Zero-order kinetics.

Each option may be used once, more than once or not at all.

Lead-in: From the following descriptions of drug clearance from the
              body, select the appropriate mechanism responsible above.

Stems: 42.1   When the clearance mechanisms of a drug are not
                     saturated, a constant fraction of that drug is cleared
                     per unit of time.

              42.2   When the clearance systems for a drug are
                     saturated, a constant amount of that drug is cleared
                     per unit of time.

              42.3   The clearance of a drug is not a linear function of its
                     blood concentration.

              42.4   The clearance of a drug is a linear function of its
                     blood concentration.

Question 43. *Early side-effects of antipsychotic treatment*

Theme: Early side-effects of antipsychotic treatment.

Options: A.   Acute dystonia.
                B.   Akathisia.
                C.   Athetosis.
                D.   Chorea.
                E.   Hemiballismus.
                F.   Parkinsonism.
                G.   Tardive dyskinesia.
                H.   Tics.
                I.   Tremors.

Each option may be used once, more than once or not at all.

Lead-in: For each of the descriptions of an acute side-effect below,
                choose the term above that best describes the following
                phenomena.

Stems: 43.1   This movement disorder occurs commonly within
                       days of exposure to an antipsychotic and is
                       inversely associated with age but positively
                       associated with the potency of the antipsychotic.

                43.2   The 'bon-bon' sign is a feature of this
                       extrapyramidal side-effect.

                43.3   This extrapyramidal side-effect occurs commonly
                       within weeks of exposure to antipsychotics and is a
                       major source of non-compliance. Its manifestation
                       has objective and subjective components.

Question 44. Mood stabilisers

Theme: Mood stabilisers.

Options: A.   Carbamazepine.
B.   Gabapentin.
C.   Lamotrigine.
D.   Leucopenia.
E.   Lithium.
F.   Neutrophilia.
G.   Thrombocytopenia.
H.   Valproate.
I.   Verapamil.

Each option may be used once, more than once or not at all.

Lead-in: For each of the following statements on the pharmacodynamics and pharmacokinetics of mood stabilisers, choose the agent/condition above that is most likely to be implicated.

Stems: 44.1   This mood stabiliser induces its own metabolism to a substantial degree. Hence after one month the initial steady-state levels may have fallen by as much as 25%.

44.2   This mood stabiliser is a powerful gastric irritant and increases lamotrigine levels.

44.3   Lithium treatment is commonly associated with this effect on blood cells during the initial phase of treatment.

44.4   Acute pancreatitis is a known complication of this mood stabiliser, as is hyperammonaemia.

Question 45. Adverse effects of the atypical antipsychotics

Theme: Adverse effects of the atypical antipsychotics.

Options: A.   Amisulpride.   E.   Quetiapine.
                     B.   Aripiprazole.   F.   Risperidone.
                     C.   Clozapine.   G.   Sertindole.
                     D.   Olanzapine.   H.   Ziprasidone.

Each option may be used once, more than once or not at all.

Lead-in: For the following patient who has experienced side-effects
                      from various atypical antipsychotics, choose the required
                      number of agents above that are most likely to have
                      caused them.

Stems: 45.1   A 24-year-old man with paranoid schizophrenia
                               complains of being unable to sit still, feeling that his
                               legs have to keep moving. He is obviously distressed
                               by this. He knows he is taking a drug for his 'voices'
                               but cannot remember the name of his medication.

                               *Which two agents from the above are the most likely
                               candidates to be the drug he is taking?*

                      45.2   He states that he had previously been tried on a
                               medication that made him feel very dizzy when he
                               stood up. He is again unsure of the name, but states
                               that he has never been on a medication that needed
                               regular blood monitoring.

                               Which agent was most likely to have been tried before?

                      45.3   He is commenced on a new atypical antipsychotic.
                               This appears to suit him better although he does
                               complain of drowsiness especially in the mornings.

                               Which medication is he most likely taking now?

Question 46. Antidepressant-related receptor and amine changes

Theme: Antidepressant-related receptor and amine changes.

Options: A.   Citalopram.
               B.   Decreases the 5-HT$_1$ receptors and increases the 5-HT$_2$ receptors.
               C.   Dopamine agonists.
               D.   Dopamine antagonists.
               E.   Increases the 5-HT$_1$ and 5-HT$_2$ receptors.
               F.   Increases the 5-HT$_1$ receptors and decreases the 5-HT$_2$ receptors.
               G.   Monoamine oxidase inhibitors.
               H.   Reduces the 5-HT$_1$ and 5-HT$_2$ receptors.
               I.   Selective serotonin reuptake inhibitors.
               J.   Tricyclics.

Each option may be used once, more than once or not at all.

Lead-in: For each of the following questions about antidepressant-related receptor and amine changes, choose the phrase above that best answers each of the following questions.

Stems: 46.1 Chronic treatment with tricyclic antidepressants causes which changes in serotonergic receptors?

               46.2 Treatment with electroconvulsive therapy (ECT) causes which changes in serotonergic receptors?

               46.3 Which group of drugs are the principal ones that modify serotonin degradation?

               46.4 Which group of drugs increase the release of serotonin?

Question 47. Anxiolytics and hypnotics

Theme: Anxiolytic and hypnotic agents.

Options: A.   Buspirone.
              B.   Chloral hydrate.
              C.   Diazepam.
              D.   Lorazepam.
              E.   Paraldehyde.
              F.   Sodium amytal.
              G.   Temazepam.
              H.   Zaleplon.
              I.   Zolpidem.
              J.   Zopiclone.

Each option may be used once, more than once or not at all.

Lead-in: From the following pharmacokinetics and pharmacodynamic effects, choose the agent above most likely to be being described.

Stems: 47.1   This agent causes headaches, possibly via its partial agonism of serotonin 5-HT$_{1A}$ receptors.

              47.2   This agent binds to the benzodiazepine-1 receptor site and has little or no hangover effect when used as a hypnotic.

              47.3   This agent has a long half-life and may be metabolised to oxazepam.

              47.4   This agent causes halitosis but is safe in individuals with impaired renal functioning.

Question 48. Adverse effects of typical antipsychotics

Theme: Adverse effects of typical antipsychotics.

Options: A.   Allergically-mediated cholestatic changes.
            B.   Both allergic reaction and direct toxicity to hepatic and biliary system.
            C.   Brightness.
            D.   Decreases in alpha waves and increases in theta and delta waves.
            E.   Decreases in alpha, theta and delta waves.
            F.   Decreased androgen levels.
            G.   Direct toxicity to the liver.
            H.   Disturbances in the oestrogen-to-androgen ratio.
            I.   Hyperprolactinaemia.
            J.   Increases in alpha waves and decreases in theta and delta waves.
            K.   Temperature.

Each option may be used once, more than once or not at all.

Lead-in: Choose the phrase above relating to adverse effects of typical antipsychotics that best relates to the following statements.

Stems: 48.1   This is the mechanism involved in producing gynaecomastia in males who are on long-term antipsychotic treatment.

          48.2   Phenothiazine-induced hepatic damage is due to this mechanism(s).

          48.3   Antipsychotic exposure causes these electroencephalogram (EEG) changes.

          48.4   To develop antipsychotic-induced photosensitivity this environmental factor is the most important.

Question 49. Psychotropic use in lactating mothers

Theme: Psychotropic use in lactating mothers.

Options: A.   Chlorpromazine.
B.   Citalopram.
C.   Clomipramine.
D.   Diazepam.
E.   Doxepin.
F.   Fluoxetine.
G.   Haloperidol.
H.   Lorazepam.
I.   Nitrazepam.
J.   Paroxetine.
K.   Sulpiride.

Each option may be used once, more than once or not at all.

Lead-in: While it is best to avoid the use of psychotropics in the lactating mother, there are times when this is necessary. Choose the drug above that is being described in the following situations.

Stems: 49.1   Even though this selective serotonin reuptake inhibitor (SSRI) is excreted in the breast milk, it is detected in infants' serum in low levels and no adverse effects have been reported.

49.2   No adverse side-effects have been reported with this tricyclic antidepressant in infants who were exposed to it by breast-feeding.

49.3   This antipsychotic has improved lactation in lactating mothers and no adverse effects were noted in the nursing infants.

49.4   This benzodiazepine is recommended for breast-feeding mothers.

Question 50. *Pharmacological profiles of the newer antidepressants*

Theme: Pharmacological profiles of the newer antidepressants.

Options: A.   Escitalopram.
               B.   Lofepramine.
               C.   Maprotiline.
               D.   Mianserin.
               E.   Mirtazapine.
               F.   Reboxetine.
               G.   Trazadone.
               H.   Venlafaxine.
               I.   Viloxazine.

Each option may be used once, more than once or not at all.

Lead-in: Choose the antidepressant above from the following
               characteristics that is most likely being described.

Stems: 50.1   This novel noradrenergic and specific serotonergic
                      antidepressant has a half-life of 20–40 hours and is
                      commonly associated with weight gain.

               50.2   This new antidepressant is structurally related to
                      fluoxetine and viloxazine. It has little inhibitory
                      effects on cytochrome P450 systems. It lacks action
                      on serotonin systems, and does not have monoamine
                      oxidase inhibitory effects.

               50.3   This antidepressant is highly sedative but has little
                      cardiac effect. It causes dry mouth but has no
                      anticholinergic effects. In the initial period it
                      requires close haematological monitoring.

Question 51. Pharmacokinetics terms

Theme: Pharmacokinetics terms.

Options:

A. Active transport.
B. Bioavailability.
C. Bioequivalence.
D. Blood–brain barrier.
E. Elimination half-life.

F. First-order kinetics.
G. First-pass effect.
H. Plasma protein binding.
I. Volume of distribution.
J. Zero-order kinetics.

Each option may be used once, more than once or not at all.

Lead-in: Each of the following situations demonstrates a concept of pharmacokinetics. Select the term above that best describes the concept.

Stems:

51.1 A given dose of morphine is much more potent when administered intravenously than when it is given orally, as the latter route of administration leads to significant amounts of the drug being inactivated rapidly.

51.2 The rate of elimination of alcohol from the body is independent of the plasma concentration of alcohol.

51.3 When chlorpromazine is given orally, only a certain amount of it is absorbed from the gastrointestinal tract. It is only the absorbed fraction that can have potential therapeutic effects.

51.4 Patients with Parkinsonism get little benefit from the administration of dopamine but they do get benefit from the administration of its precursor, levo-dopa.

Question 52. Commencing clozapine treatment

Theme:　　Commencing clozapine treatment.

Options:　　A.　　Admit to hospital.
　　　　　　　B.　　Check creatinine kinase.
　　　　　　　C.　　Check full blood count.
　　　　　　　D.　　Prescribe an antipyretic.
　　　　　　　E.　　Prescribe hyoscine.
　　　　　　　F.　　Prescribe sulpiride.
　　　　　　　G.　　Reduce titration rate.
　　　　　　　H.　　Refer to a cardiologist.
　　　　　　　I.　　Stop clozapine therapy.
　　　　　　　J.　　Take no action.

Each option may be used once, more than once or not at all.

Lead-in:　　David is a 28-year-old unemployed builder with treatment-resistant paranoid schizophrenia. He has agreed to commencement of clozapine therapy on a day hospital-attendee basis. Read the following questions and select the required number of options above as answers.

Stems:　　52.1　　The patient notices marked salivation in the first two weeks of initiation, such that his pillow is saturated when he wakes in the morning. *What action from the above would you choose?*

　　　　　　52.2　　During the third week of initiation, one of the day hospital nurses informs you that the patient's temperature is 38.5°C. *What two actions from the above would you choose?*

　　　　　　52.3　　During the fifth week of initiation, the nurse informs you that the patient has an increased heart rate of 105/minute that seems to have persisted over the last few weeks and which is associated with a blood pressure that frequently falls to 80/50 mmHg. *What action from the above would you choose?*

　　　　　　52.4　　The above step reassures you and titration proceeds. A full blood count in the sixth week of initiation reveals that the patient has a markedly reduced neutrophil count. *What two actions from the above would you choose?*

Question 53. Adverse effects of antidepressants

Theme: Adverse effects of antidepressants.

Options: A.   Amitriptyline.   G.   Lofepramine.
             B.   Citalopram.   H.   Phenelzine.
             C.   Clomipramine.   I.   Reboxetine.
             D.   Doxepin.   J.   Sertraline.
             E.   Fluoxetine.   K.   Trazodone.
             F.   Imipramine.   L.   Venlafaxine.

Each option may be used once, more than once or not at all.

Lead-in: For each patient, select the antidepressant most likely to have caused the side-effect.

Stems: 53.1   A 36-year-old woman on antidepressant therapy develops sweating, nausea, headache and a stiff neck acutely, after using an over-the-counter preparation containing ephedrine.

         53.2   A 24-year-old man, commenced recently on a selective serotonin reuptake inhibitor, develops headache and reduced appetite.

         53.3   A 72-year-old woman dies following an intentional overdose of her antidepressant tablets.

         53.4   A 56-year-old man on antidepressant therapy complains of drowsiness during the day.

Question 54. *Pharmacology of pregnancy and the puerperium*

Theme: Pharmacology of pregnancy and the puerperium.

Options: A.   Fluoxetine.   F.   Paroxetine.
               B.   Haloperidol.   G.   Sulpiride.
               C.   Lofepramine.   H.   Trifluoperazine.
               D.   Moclobemide.   I.   Zolpidem.
               E.   Olanzapine.   J.   Zopiclone.

Each option may be used once, more than once or not at all.

Lead-in: For each of the following women, select the agent above
               that is most appropriate for the treatment of her
               symptoms. Assume that the benefits of pharmacotherapy
               outweigh the disadvantages.

Stems: 54.1   A 23-year-old woman in the first trimester of
                      pregnancy develops agitation, paranoid ideation and
                      third person auditory hallucinations. Her appetite,
                      energy and sleep are all normal.

               54.2   A 31-year-old woman in the second trimester of
                      pregnancy develops low mood, hopelessness and
                      suicidal ideation. Her appetite, energy and sleep are
                      all reduced.

               54.3   A 31-year-old woman who is breastfeeding her one-
                      month-old infant develops low mood, hopelessness
                      and suicidal ideation. Her appetite, energy and
                      sleep are all reduced.

               54.4   A 27-year-old woman who is breastfeeding her two-
                      month-old infant develops severe sleep disturbance
                      but has no other symptoms of psychiatric illness.

Question 55. *Choice of antidepressants*

Theme: Choice of antidepressants.

Options: A.   Amitriptyline.
B.   Clomipramine.
C.   Dothiepin.
D.   Escitalopram.
E.   Fluoxetine.
F.   Fluvoxamine.
G.   ,Moclobemide.
H.   Paroxetine.
I.   Phenelzine.
J.   Tranylcypromine.

Each option may be used once, more than once or not at all.

Lead-in: A 40-year-old female has a three-month history of low mood, decreased energy, poor appetite, early morning waking and thoughts of self-harm.

Read the following questions and select the required antidepressant above.

Stems: 55.1   The woman is worried about becoming dependent on antidepressants.

Which antidepressant is most likely to cause dependence?

55.2   Since she has had a history of rashes on medication before, you are keen to select an antidepressant that is less likely to cause a rash.

Which antidepressant is most likely to cause a rash?

55.3   She has a degree in pharmacology and asks you about active metabolites of antidepressants.

Which antidepressant has weak metabolites?

55.4   It appears she developed her depression on a background of long-standing generalised anxiety disorder.

Which agent is licensed for the treatment of generalised anxiety disorder?

Question 56. Drugs of use in substance misuse treatment

Theme: Drugs of use in substance misuse treatment.

Options: A.   Acamprosate.   F.   Diazepam.
                B.   Buprenorphine.   G.   Disulfiram.
                C.   Chlordiazepoxide.   H.   Lofexidine.
                D.   Clonidine.   I.   Methadone.
                E.   Clomethiazole.   J.   Naltrexone.

Each option may be used once, more than once or not at all.

Lead-in: For each of the following patients on treatment for
                substance misuse, choose the agent above that is most
                likely to be responsible for their symptoms.

Stems: 56.1   A 36-year-old man with alcohol dependence is
                       commenced on a medication for his dependence
                       following detoxification. His clinical team is aware
                       that he still abuses alcohol on an intermittent basis.
                       The main symptoms he experiences while on this
                       medication are a transient rash, mild diarrhoea and
                       some variation in his libido.

                       *On which medication was he most likely to be
                       commenced?*

                56.2   A 56-year-old woman is receiving ongoing
                       medication for the last four months. When she takes
                       some cough suppressant she bought over the
                       counter she develops severe nausea and headache
                       along with flushing of her face. When she stands up
                       she feels faint and almost falls over.

                       What medication was she taking for the last four months?

                56.3   A 21-year-old man is being treated for withdrawal
                       symptoms. He complains of pallor and pain in his
                       fingers when they are exposed to the cold. The pain
                       worsens when he tries to warm his fingers over the
                       fire.

                       Which medication is he most likely to be taking?

Question 57. *Effects of antidepressants on receptors*

Theme: Effects of antidepressants on receptors.

Options: A. α_1-adrenoreceptor.
B. α_1-adrenoreceptor and histamine H_1-receptor.
C. α_1-adrenoreceptor and muscarinic receptor.
D. α_1-adrenoreceptor and serotonergic receptor.
E. Histamine H_1-receptor.
F. Histamine H_1-receptor and muscarinic receptor.
G. Histamine H_1-receptor and serotonergic receptor.
H. Muscarinic receptor and serotonergic receptor.
I. Serotonergic receptor and dopaminergic receptor.
J. Serotonergic receptor and β_2-adrenoreceptor.

Each option may be used once, more than once or not at all.

Lead-in: A 32-year-old male has a five-month history of ICD-10 depressive disorder of moderate severity with somatic symptoms associated with moderate suicidal risk. He responded only to amitriptyline. Choose the receptor(s) above *most likely* to have been acted directly upon to cause the following effects.

Stems: 57.1 He feels dizzy when he stands up.

57.2 He complains of drowsiness.

57.3 He notes he has gained half a stone in weight.

57.4 He confides that his sexual performance is impaired.

Question 58. *Pharmacokinetics and pharmacodynamics of the benzodiazepines*

Theme: Pharmacokinetics and pharmacodynamics of the benzodiazepines.

Options: A.   Active metabolite of lorazepam has a longer half-life.
               B.   Anterograde amnesia.
               C.   Both anterograde and retrograde amnesia.
               D.   Both by increasing the number of channels opened and prolonging the duration of channel opening.
               E.   Increasing the number of channels opened.
               F.   Prolonging the duration of the opening of the channels.
               G.   Rapid degradation of diazepam.
               H.   Retrograde amnesia.
               I.   Slow and less-wide distribution of lorazepam.

Each option may be used once, more than once or not at all.

Lead-in: Choose the phrase above that best fits the following statements on the actions of the benzodiazepines.

Stems: 58.1   Benzodiazepines facilitate γ-aminobutyric acid (GABA) inhibition by this action on the chloride channels.

             58.2   Intravenous lorazepam has a longer action than intravenous diazepam because of this reason.

             58.3   Controlled studies have shown that benzodiazepines produce this form of amnesia.

Question 59. *Side-effects of antidepressants*

Theme: Side-effects of antidepressants.

Options: A. Amitriptyline.   G. L-tryptophan.
               B. Citalopram.   H. Maprotiline.
               C. Clomipramine.   I. Mirtazapine.
               D. Fluoxetine.   J. Nortriptyline.
               E. Fluvoxamine.   K. Phenelzine.
               F. Imipramine.   L. Venlafaxine.

Each option may be used once, more than once or not at all.

Lead-in: For each patient below, select the antidepressant above
               that is most likely to have caused the side-effect.

Stems: 59.1 A 47-year-old woman has been on antidepressant
               therapy for two years. A week after the dose of
               medication has been increased because of symptom
               recurrence she has a seizure for the first time in her
               life.

               59.2 A 32-year-old man has to have his antidepressant
               medication discontinued because of disabling
               sedation.

               59.3 A 51-year-old man stops taking his prescribed
               antidepressants after five days because of
               intolerable vomiting.

               59.4 A 63-year-old woman has been on antidepressant
               therapy for over ten years. She complains of tingling
               sensation in her feet and has areas of numbness
               there as well.

Question 60. *Pharmacodynamics of anxiolytic medications*

Theme: Pharmacodynamics of anxiolytic medications.

Options: A.   Alprazolam.   E.   Clobazam.
              B.   Bromazepam.   F.   Diazepam.
              C.   Buspirone.   G.   Lorazepam.
              D.   Chlordiazepoxide.   H.   Propranolol.

Each option may be used once, more than once or not at all.

Lead-in: From the following descriptions of patients with anxiety
              symptoms, choose the required number of agents above
              most likely to have caused the indicated effects.

Stems: 60.1   A 37-year-old housewife with panic disorder runs
                     out of her prescription of anxiolytic on a regular
                     basis. Rather than face censure from her own
                     general practitioner, she visits a number of different
                     doctors on such occasions to get the prescription
                     renewed. *(Choose one option)*

              60.2   A 53-year-old man with generalised anxiety
                     disorder complains of somnolence, which he
                     correctly attributes to his medication. *(Choose three
                     options)*

              60.3   A 35-year-old man with hepatic impairment
                     develops agoraphobia and is prescribed a short
                     course of a benzodiazepine by his psychiatrist
                     before commencing a selective serotonin reuptake
                     inhibitor. *(Choose one option)*

              60.4   A 62-year-old woman with generalised anxiety
                     disorder develops a heart rate of 100 beats per
                     minute after being commenced on an anxiolytic.
                     (Choose one option)

Question 61. Lithium

Theme: Lithium.

Options: A.   Daily divided dose.
 B.   Duodenum.
 C.   Large bowel when the water content is greater.
 D.   Large bowel when the water content is less.
 E.   Single nighttime dose.
 F.   Small bowel by active transport.
 G.   Small bowel by passive diffusion.
 H.   Stomach irrespective of pH levels.
 I.   Stomach when the pH is high.
 J.   Stomach when the pH is low.

Each option may be used once, more than once or not at all.

Lead-in: Choose the phrase above that best answers each of the
 following questions on the pharmacokinetics of lithium.

Stems: 61.1   Where does the absorption of lithium
 predominantly occur?

 61.2   When lithium concentrations are high in the
 gastrointestinal tract, where is absorption fastest?

 61.3   What is the second most important site for lithium
 absorption?

 61.4   Which dosing regimen results in peak levels of
 plasma lithium twice those of trough levels?

Question 62. *Pharmacodynamics of hypnotic agents*

Theme: Pharmacodynamics of hypnotic agents.

Options: A.   Chloral betane.   E.   Temazepam.
                 B.   Flunitrazepam.   F.   Zaleplon.
                 C.   Nitrazepam.   G.   Zolpidem.
                 D.   Promethazine.   H.   Zopiclone.

Each option may be used once, more than once or not at all.

Lead-in: From the following descriptions of patients who are taking
                 a hypnotic, choose the agent above most likely to have
                 caused the indicated effects.

Stems: 62.1   A 71-year-old man refuses to consider a gradual
                        reduction in his hypnotic because he says he tried
                        this a number of times over the years and has
                        always suffered marked symptoms such as
                        insomnia, nightmares, increased anxiety and
                        sweating as a result.

                 62.2   A 59-year-old woman complains of severe nausea
                        while taking a prescribed hypnotic.

                 62.3   A 35-year-old woman asks her general practitioner
                        for a change in hypnotic as she finds herself drowsy
                        in the morning and finds it difficult to function at
                        work for the first few hours.

                 62.4   A 28-year-old male complains of a metallic taste
                        after commencing a hypnotic medication.

Question 63. Antidepressants: adverse effects

Theme: Antidepressants: adverse effects.

Options: A.   Anticholinergic action.
B.   Both α_1-adrenergic antagonism and anticholinergic actions.
C.   Both by suppressing sino-atrial node functions and delaying ventricular conduction time.
D.   Both central and local actions on the gastrointestinal system.
E.   Central mechanisms that control gastrointestinal functions.
F.   Delaying ventricular conduction time.
G.   Fluoxetine.
H.   Local actions on the gastrointestinal system.
I.   Paroxetine.
J.   Potent α_1-adrenergic antagonism.

Each option may be used once, more than once or not at all.

Lead-in: Antidepressant drugs are associated with a wide range of adverse effects. Some drugs produce more adverse effects than others, even those belonging to the same chemical group. The mechanism involved in producing those effects can be associated with certain actions of a drug or group of drugs.

Choose the option above that most closely fits the following statements.

Stems: 63.1   Trazodone produces dry mouth and blurred vision because of its action on this receptor(s).

63.2   Selective serotonin reuptake inhibitor (SSRI) induced gastrointestinal upsets are likely to be mediated by these actions.

63.3   At high blood levels tricyclic antidepressants cause ventricular tachyarrhythmias due to this action on the heart.

63.4   A discontinuation syndrome is relatively uncommon following the cessation of this SSRI.

Question 64. Anticholinergic drugs

Theme: Anticholinergic drugs.

Options: A.   Benzhexol.   E.   Orphenadrine.
               B.   Benztropine.   F.   Pirenzepine.
               C.   Biperiden.   G.   Procyclidine.
               D.   Hyoscine.   H.   Tetrabenazine.

Each option may be used once, more than once or not at all.

Lead-in: For each of the following patients, select the
               anticholinergic agent above he/she is most likely to be
               using.

Stems: 64.1   A 23-year-old man with schizophrenia has fixed
                       dilated pupils. He states that he lost his last
                       prescription and wants you to give him another for
                       his anticholinergic medication because he feels they
                       help his depression.

               64.2   A 68-year-old woman with treatment-resistant
                       depression kills herself by taking an overdose of her
                       son's anticholinergic tablets.

               64.3   A 56-year-old woman with schizophrenia develops a
                       depressive episode. When a monoamine oxidase
                       inhibitor is added to her treatment, she becomes
                       acutely confused.

Question 65. *Anticonvulsant agents*

Theme: Anticonvulsant agents.

Options:

A.	Carbamazepine.	F.	Phenobarbitone.
B.	Clonazepam.	G.	Phenytoin.
C.	Gabapentin.	H.	Sodium valproate.
D.	Ethosuximide.	I.	Topiramate.
E.	Lamotrigine.	J.	Vigabatrin.

Each option may be used once, more than once or not at all.

Lead-in: For each of the following patients, select the anticonvulsant agent above that is most likely to be causing his/her side-effects.

Stems: 65.1 A 47-year-old woman with bipolar affective disorder develops a rash while taking her anticonvulsant mood stabiliser. She also complains of headache and, on liver function tests, is found to have raised enzymes.

65.2 A 36-year-old woman with a history of partial seizures complains of difficulties with her memory and of sedation. Blood tests are unremarkable but she reports being pleased that she has lost 3 kg in weight recently.

65.3 A 29-year-old man with temporal lobe epilepsy was started on a new anticonvulsant because of treatment refractory seizures. He developed a new-onset psychotic episode two months after commencing therapy, and has recently been found to have reduced peripheral vision. Blood tests are unremarkable.

65.4 A 31-year-old man with learning difficulties and generalised tonic-clonic seizures is noted to be ataxic and sedated. A full blood count reveals a folate-deficient anaemia.

Question 66. *Pharmacodynamics of antidepressants*

Theme: Pharmacodynamics of antidepressants.

Options: A.   Adrenaline α_1-receptor.
                B.   Adrenaline α_2-receptor.
                C.   Dopamine D_2-receptor.
                D.   Dopamine reuptake pump.
                E. $GABA_A$ receptor.
                F.   Histamine H_1-receptor.
                G.   Muscarine M_1-receptor.
                H.   Noradrenaline reuptake pump.
                I.   Serotonin 5-HT_2-receptor.
                J.   Serotonin 5-HT_3-receptor.
                K.   Serotonin 5-HT_7-receptor.
                L.   Serotonin reuptake pump.

Each option may be used once, more than once or not at all.

Lead-in: For each of the following antidepressants, select the
                required number of receptors from the list above that are
                most characteristically acted upon by the drug.

Stems: 66.1   Venlafaxine. *(Select three responses)*

                66.2   Mirtazapine. *(Select four responses)*

                66.3   Fluoxetine. *(Select three responses)*

                66.4   Bupropion. *(Select two responses)*

Question 67. *Pharmacodynamics of anti-manic agents*

Theme: Pharmacodynamics of anti-manic agents.

Options: A.   Carbamazepine.
                B.   Clonazepam.
                C.   Gabapentin.
                D.   Lamotrigine.
                E.   Lithium carbonate.
                F.   Olanzapine.
                G.   Risperidone.
                H.   Sodium valproate.
                I.   Topiramate.
                J.   Verapamil.

Each option may be used once, more than once or not at all.

Lead-in: Select the agent above that matches each of the following
                pharmacodynamic profiles.

Stems: 67.1 Entry of cells via sodium channels and inhibition of
                      the phosphoinositide second messenger system.

                67.2 Interference with sodium and calcium channels
                      thereby enhancing the function of GABA and
                      reducing that of glutamate. Also, inhibition of
                      carbonic anhydrase.

                67.3 Inhibition of cAMP production and potentiation of
                      serotonin (5-HT) responses by increasing 5-HT
                      release and increasing 5-HT receptor sensitivity.

Question 68. Impairment of glucose tolerance and atypical antipsychotics

Theme: Impairment of glucose tolerance and atypical antipsychotics.

Options: A.   Amisulpiride.
                B.   Aripiprazole.
                C.   Clozapine.
                D.   Olanzapine.
                E.   Quetiapine.
                F.   Risperidone.
                G.   Ziprasidone.

Each option may be used once, more than once or not at all.

Lead-in: Hyperglycaemia is strongly linked to treatment with both conventional and atypical antipsychotics. Select the atypical antipsychotic above to which each of the following statements most likely refers.

Stems: 68.1   This atypical antipsychotic has been strongly associated with hyperglycaemia, impaired glucose tolerance and diabetic ketoacidosis. Most cases of diabetes are noted in the first six months of treatment. A third of patients may develop diabetes after five years of treatment with this drug.

                68.2   This atypical antipsychotic has been strongly linked to impaired glucose tolerance, diabetes and diabetic ketoacidosis, but the time course of development of diabetes has not been established.

                68.3   Combining this atypical with clozapine may ameliorate clozapine-related diabetes.

Question 69. Drug interactions

Theme: Drug interactions.

Options: A. Amiloride.
B. Frusemide.
C. Gin.
D. Ibuprofen.
E. Insulin.
F. Paracetamol.
G. Paraldehyde.
H. Phenylpropanolamine.
I. Tetracycline.
J. Warfarin.

Each option may be used once, more than once or not at all.

Lead-in: For each of the following patients, **select two** of the agents above that are most likely to have caused the interaction with their current pharmacotherapy.

Stems: 69.1 A 56-year-old woman with recurrent depression has been taking phenelzine for years. After taking another agent, she develops severe nausea, sweating and headache and her blood pressure is later found to be markedly elevated.

69.2 A 37-year-old man with bipolar affective disorder has been stabilised on lithium treatment. After taking another agent, he develops nausea, a coarse tremor and slurring of speech.

69.3 A 53-year-old woman with alcohol dependence has been commenced on disulfiram. After taking another agent, she develops severe headache, nausea and flushing and her blood pressure is found to be lowered.

69.4 A 20-year-old man with heroin addiction is receiving maintenance methadone treatment. After taking another agent, he develops marked drowsiness and respiratory depression.

Question 70. *Monoamine oxidase inhibitors*

Theme: Monoamine oxidase inhibitors (MAOIs).

Options: A.   Both postural and supine hypotension.
                B.   Continue the same dose.
                C.   Cottage cheese.
                D.   Late in treatment.
                E.   *Liederkrantz* blue cheese.
                F.   Over the first four weeks.
                G.   Postural hypotension only.
                H.   Reduce the dose.
                I.   Stop the drug.
                J.   Supine hypotension only.

Each option may be used once, more than once or not at all.

Lead-in: A 50-year-old woman has a history of atypical depression.
                She has responded to tranylcypromine but not to other
                antidepressants. Select the option above that most closely
                matches each of the following statements about MAOI
                therapy.

Stems: 70.1   She is likely to have this type(s) of medication-
                      related hypotension.

              70.2   The postural hypotension commonly manifests
                      during this period after the initiation of treatment.

              70.3   The woman has developed cirrhosis of the liver. In
                      this situation one should follow this strategy with
                      regard to antidepressant treatment.

              70.4   The woman must avoid using this milk product in
                      her food.

Question 71. Drugs in dementia.

Theme: Use of pharmacological agents in the dementias.

Options:

A.	Choline.	F.	Nicotinic acid.
B.	Donepezil.	G.	Physostigmine.
C.	Galanthamine.	H.	Rivastigmine.
D.	*Ginkgo biloba.*	I.	Tacrine.
E.	Lecithin.	J.	Tyrosine.

Each option may be used once, more than once or not at all.

Lead-in: Select the required number of agents above that best fit the descriptions of putative modes of action in dementia below.

Stems: 71.1 Patients with Alzheimer's disease are thought to have reduced antioxidant activity, leading to the trial of drugs with antioxidant activity. (Select one item)

71.2 Atherosclerosis of cerebral blood vessels was hypothesized to create or compound cognitive decline, hence the use of agents with vasodilatory action. (Select one item)

71.3 Since Alzheimer's disease has been found extensively to be associated with reduced cerebral acetylcholine, administration of precursors of this neurotransmitter might be expected to improve cholinergic activity. (Select two items)

71.4 Agents that inhibit acetylcholinesterase relatively selectively over pseudocholinesterase are thought to be effective in Alzheimer's disease since they reduce the breakdown of acetylcholine and acetylcholinesterase is the key enzyme for this at cholinergic synapses. (Select four items)

Question 72. Side-effects of the newer antidepressants

Theme: Side-effects of the newer antidepressants.

Options: A. Anorexia.
                B. Constipation.
                C. Diarrhoea.
                D. Dizziness.
                E. Drowsiness.
                F. Dry mouth.
                G. Fine tremor.
                H. Headache.
                I. Insomnia.
                J. Nausea.
                K. Nervousness.
                L. Weight gain.

Each option may be used once, more than once or not at all.

Lead-in: For each of the following antidepressants, select the
                required number of its most common side-effects above
                (compared to rates on placebo) reported by patients.

Stems: 72.1   Fluoxetine. *(Select two items)*

                72.2   Reboxetine. *(Select three items)*

                72.3   Venlafaxine. *(Select two items)*

                72.4   Mirtazapine. *(Select three items)*

Question 73. Side-effects of antipsychotics

Theme: Side-effects of antipsychotics.

Options: A.   Amisulpride.   F.   Haloperidol.
               B.   Chlorpromazine.   G.   Pimozide.
               C.   Clozapine.   H.   Quetiapine.
               D.   Flupenthixol.   I.   Risperidone.
               E.   Fluphenazine.   J.   Thioridazine.

Each option may be used once, more than once or not at all.

Lead-in: For each of the following patients on antipsychotic
              therapy, select the agent most likely to have caused
              his/her side-effects.

Stems: 73.1   A 56-year-old woman complains of feeling
                    groggy in the morning and tired through the
                    day. She has a marked tremor with cogwheel
                    rigidity at the wrists. There are no
                    abnormalities on electrocardiogram (ECG).
                    She has gained 3 kg in weight since
                    commencing therapy. She has frequent
                    constipation and blurring of vision.

            73.2   A 32-year-old man denies feeling tired
                    during the day. He notes some restlessness in
                    his legs, but only finds this mildly troubling,
                    and he has cogwheel rigidity at the wrists. He
                    is noted to have a prolonged QTc interval on
                    ECG. He has not gained any weight since
                    commencing therapy. He denies any
                    constipation or blurring of vision.

            73.3   A 27-year-old woman complains of feeling
                    tired, particularly in the mornings. There is
                    no evidence of tremor or cogwheel rigidity.
                    There are non-significant ECG changes. She
                    has gained 6 kg in weight since commencing
                    therapy. She notes frequent constipation and
                    some blurring of vision.

Question 74. Signs of lithium toxicity

Theme: Signs of lithium toxicity.

Options: A.   Apathy.   G.   Polydipsia.
               B.   Coarse tremor.   H.   Poor concentration.
               C.   Diarrhoea.   I.   Severe fine tremor.
               D.   Disorientation.   J.   Slurred speech.
               E.   Fine tremor.   K.   Spasticity.
               F.   Incontinence.   L.   Vomiting.

Each option may be used once only.

Lead-in: For each of the following levels of lithium toxicity, select
               the required number of the most appropriate side-effects
               or toxicity signs above that are *particularly* associated with
               that level.

Stems: 74.1   A 36-year-old man with bipolar affective disorder
                      on lithium therapy has no signs of lithium toxicity.

                      Select three side-effects he may be experiencing.

               74.2   A 78-year-old woman receiving lithium
                      augmentation therapy develops mild lithium
                      toxicity.

                      *Select two toxicity signs she may be experiencing. You may
                      not choose any options you have already used.*

               74.3   A 45-year-old woman being treated with lithium for
                      acute mania develops moderate lithium toxicity.

                      *Select four toxicity signs she may be experiencing. You may
                      not choose any options you have already used.*

               74.4   A 23-year-old man with borderline personality
                      disorder overdoses on a friend's lithium tablets and
                      develops severe lithium toxicity.

                      *Select three toxicity signs he may be experiencing. You may
                      not choose any options you have already used.*

Descriptive and Psychodynamic Psychopathology EMIs

Question 75. Defence mechanisms

Theme: Defence mechanisms.

Options:
A.	Acting out.	G.	Rationalization.
B.	Denial.	H.	Reaction formation.
C.	Displacement.	I.	Repression.
D.	Idealization.	J.	Sublimation.
E.	Projection.	K.	Suppression.
F.	Projective identification.	L.	Undoing.

Each option may be used once, more than once or not at all.

Lead-in: For each of the following, choose the term above that most closely describes the main defence mechanism employed by the individual.

Stems:

75.1 A man habitually deals with upsetting events by deciding not to think about them.

75.2 A girl who has repetitive distressing thoughts of harming her family follows occurrences of these thoughts by repeating a short phrase that she hopes protects them.

75.3 A woman with alcohol problems states that she would be able to give up drinking quite easily if her husband would only stop tormenting her and instead pay more attention to her.

75.4 A man with marked aggressive impulses takes up rugby as a pastime.

Question 76. Individuals associated with psychopathological syndromes

Theme: Individuals associated with psychopathological syndromes.

Options: A.   Agoraphobia.
                B.   Anaclitic depression.
                C.   Anankastic personality.
                D.   Anorexia nervosa.
                E.   Bulimia nervosa.
                F.   Catatonic schizophrenia.
                G.   Dementia praecox.
                H.   Dysthymia.
                I.   Munchausen syndrome.
                J.   Neurasthenia.
                K.   Schizoaffective disorder.
                L.   Schizophreniform psychosis.

Each option may be used once, more than once or not at all.

Lead-in: For each of the following individuals, choose the syndrome
                he/she is most associated with above.

Stems: 76.1   Kraepelin.

                76.2   Kahlbaum.

                76.3   Beard.

                76.4   Gull.

Question 77. *Psychopathological syndromes*

Theme: Psychopathological syndromes.

Options: A. Briquet's syndrome.
         B. Capgras' syndrome.
         C. Charles Bonnet syndrome.
         D. Cotard's syndrome.
         E. Couvade syndrome.
         F. De Clérambault
             syndrome.

         G. Ekbom's syndrome.
         H. Frégoli syndrome.
         I. Ganser syndrome.
         J. Meadow's syndrome.
         K. Othello syndrome.
         L. Pickwickian
             syndrome.

Each option may be used once at most.

Lead-in: For each of the following patients pick the
         psychopathological syndrome above that best describes
         his/her condition.

Stems: 77.1   A 21-year-old woman is referred after an
             altercation with a stranger. The patient states that,
             although this stranger looked perfectly ordinary, he
             was in fact former US President Bill Clinton. The
             patient believes that he has been stalking her for a
             number of months; however, others do not
             recognise him as he assumes a number of disguises.

         77.2   A 78-year-old woman is admitted with signs of
             severe psychomotor retardation. Despite being
             visited regularly by her children, she states that she
             has no family. She also believes that her bowels
             'have turned to dust'.

         77.3   A 24-year-old mother brings her 30-month-old
             child to accident & emergency stating that she has
             noticed frank blood in the child's urine. A review of
             the chart reveals they have attended the hospital
             twenty times in the last year with a variety of
             complaints and have been seen by almost all
             specialities. However, no specific pathology has
             been documented to date.

         77.4   A 33-year-old man presents to his general
             practitioner complaining of abdominal pains and
             vomiting in the mornings. Despite thorough
             investigation there appears to be no physical basis
             for these symptoms. The man is very worried about
             his wife being three months pregnant but strongly
             denies thinking that he is pregnant himself.

Question 78. Disturbance of mood

Theme: Disturbance of mood.

Options:
    A.   Anxiety.
    B.   Depression.
    C.   Females.
    D.   Females and males.
    E.   Inverse correlation.
    F.   Irritability.
    G.   Males.
    H.   No correlation.
    I.   Obsessive compulsive disorder.
    J.   Positive correlation.
    K.   Puerperal mood disorder.

Each option may be used once, more than once or not at all.

Lead-in: A 25-year-old female was distressed, since she could not control her temper and this resulted in her swearing at her relatives frequently. Choose the term above that best answers each of the following questions on disturbances of mood.

Stems:
    78.1   Which mood disturbance listed above is most likely to be responsible for her mental state?

    78.2   This mental state is particularly common in which clinical condition listed above?

    78.3   The severity of this mental state is most likely to be correlated with age in which way?

    78.4   In which gender(s) does this mental state typically occur?

Question 79. *Employment of defence mechanisms*

Theme: Employment of defence mechanisms.

Options: A.   Conversion.
               B.   Displacement.
               C.   Dissociation.
               D.   Idealisation.
               E.   Introjection.
               F.   Projection.
               G.   Rationalisation.
               H.   Reaction formation.
               I.   Regression.
               J.   Sublimation.

Each option may be used once, more than once or not at all.

Lead-in: The situations given below are the manifestation of using which one of the above defence mechanisms?

Stems: 79.1   A line manager, to whom his immediate superior was verbally aggressive, behaved in a verbally aggressive manner to his subordinate.

               79.2   A senior house officer, who has to give up psychiatry because he exhausted all of his attempts at Part I, tells himself that psychiatry is a rubbish discipline anyway.

               79.3   A man, who has repressed impulses to flirt with other men, accuses his girlfriend of flirting without having any evidence to substantiate it.

               79.4   A seven-year-old child who has achieved bladder control has developed bed wetting again following the birth of a younger sibling.

Question 80. *Delusional beliefs*

Theme: Delusional beliefs.

Options: A.   Delusion of doubles.   G.   Made feelings.
               B.   Delusion of grandeur.   H.   Nihilistic delusion.
               C.   Delusion of infidelity.   I.   Primary delusion.
               D.   Delusion of poverty.   J.   Querulant delusion.
               E.   Delusion of reference.   K.   Somatic passivity.
               F.   Erotomania.   L.   Thought insertion.

Each option may be used once, more than once or not at all.

Lead-in: For each of the following patients, select the term above
               that most closely describes his/her delusional belief.

Stems: 80.1   A 78-year-old woman with a history of bipolar
                     affective disorder scandalises her local village by
                     stating that she and the postman are having an
                     affair. The postman, some forty years her junior, is
                     at pains to deny this accusation to everyone,
                     particularly his wife.

             80.2   A 37-year-old woman with a history of
                    schizophrenia attends psychiatric outpatients.
                    While she refuses to take medication, she feels it is
                    good to talk about the trauma she encountered by
                    having to leave home because her husband had
                    been replaced by an impostor who looked exactly
                    the same, except for having larger genitals.

             80.3   A 65-year-old man with a history of recurrent
                    depression refuses to be referred to a
                    gastroenterologist by his general practitioner for
                    altered bowel habit. He feels that the suggestion is
                    pointless since he has had no organs left in his
                    abdomen for the last year and a half.

             80.4   A 23-year-old man with no previous psychiatric
                    history denies suffering from depression despite
                    reports from other family members. He accepts that
                    he looks sad and is tearful, but states that the cast
                    of the TV soap opera, *Eastenders*, are using devices
                    connected to the television cameras to cause him to
                    feel depressed.

Question 81. Disorders of movement and behaviour

Theme: Disorders of movement and behaviour.

Options: A.   Agitation.
B.   *Flexibilitas cerea.*
C.   Hyperactivity.
D.   Negativism.
E.   Obstruction.
F.   Resistance.
G.   *Schnauzkrampf.*
H.   Stereotypy.
I.   Tics.

Each option may be used once, more than once or not at all.

Lead-in: For each of the following individuals, choose the disturbance of movement or behaviour above that is most likely to be present.

Stems: 81.1   A 55-year-old female is feeling mentally restless and this causes increased arousal and physical restlessness for her.

81.2   A 32-year-old male, while carrying out a motor act, stopped still for a while and then continued his act. He cannot account for pausing his act.

81.3   A 22-year-old has an unusual facial expression in which his nose and lips are drawn together in a pout.

81.4   A 19-year-old male sits facing away from the interviewer.

Question 82. Psychopathological features of severe depression

Theme: Psychopathological features of severe depression.

Options: A.   Anergia.   F.   Depressive stupor.
              B.   Anhedonia.   G.   Derealization.
              C.   Delusion of guilt.   H.   Intropunitive.
              D.   Delusion of poverty.   I.   Nihilistic delusion.
              E.   Depersonalisation.   J.   Psychomotor retardation.

Each option may be used once, more than once or not at all.

Lead-in: Each of the following patients has severe depression.
              Choose the term above that best describes what each is
              experiencing.

Stems: 82.1   A 72-year-old man believes that he is in danger of
                    imminent arrest by the police for paedophilia
                    despite having never committed such a crime.

            82.2   A 63-year-old woman states with conviction that
                    the universe has ceased to exist.

            82.3   A 53-year-old woman takes twenty minutes to rise
                    from her chair. When she is questioned about this it
                    takes her three minutes to respond in a slow,
                    monotonous voice.

            82.4   A 28-year-old man has great difficulty describing
                    how he is feeling. He feels as if he has changed,
                    feeling as if he is a mannequin, a pale shadow of his
                    former self.

Question 83. Bipolar affective disorder and perceptual abnormalities

Theme: Bipolar affective disorder and perceptual abnormalities.

Options: A.   Command hallucination.
B.   Complex hallucination.
C.   Dysmegalopsia.
D.   Elementary hallucination.
E.   Illusion.
F.   Macropsia.
G.   Pareidolic illusion.
H.   Running commentary voices.
I.   Second person voices.
J.   Visual hyperaesthesia.

Each option may be used once, more than once or not at all.

Lead-in: A 55-year-old man has a 15-year history of bipolar affective disorder. During a recent review, he gives a history of the following experiences. For each of these, choose the psychopathological term above that best describes his experience.

Stems: 83.1   Colours appear to him to be brighter and more vivid than usual.

83.2   He believes that there is a threat to kill him. He perceives a wooden stick as a gun.

83.3   He hears low whirring noises.

83.4   Voices are telling him that he is the saviour of the world. (Select two items)

Question 84. Psychopathological features of anxiety-related states.

Theme: Psychopathological features of anxiety-related states.

Options: A. Agitation.   F. Irritability.
               B. Avoidance.   G. Obsessional impulse.
               C. Compulsive checking.   H. Obsessional rumination.
               D. Compulsive image.   I. Panic attack.
               E. Free-floating anxiety.   J. Situational anxiety.

Each option may be used once, more than once or not at all.

Lead-in: For each of the following patients with anxiety-related symptoms, chose the term above that most closely represents his/her experience.

Stems: 84.1   A teenager always screams when she sees a mouse.

               84.2   A middle-aged woman looks scared and has a furrowed brow. When asked about what is worrying her, she looks perplexed and says: 'Oh – anything and everything, nothing really.'

               84.3   A young man is distressed by the recurrent urge he gets to shout aloud a score out of ten whenever he sees a pretty girl.

               84.4   A middle-aged man feels marked anxiety that has come on unexpectedly. This anxiety reaches a crescendo within minutes and fades away shortly afterwards. He feels his heart beating and notices increased sweating and pins and needles in his fingers.

Question 85. *Formal thought disorder*

Theme: Formal thought disorder.

Options:
    A.   Circumstantiality.
    B.   Clang association.
    C.   Depression.
    D.   Derailment.
    E.   Flight of ideas.
    F.   Mania.
    G.   Neologism.
    H.   Panic disorder.
    I.   Perseveration.
    J.   Tangentiality.

Each option may be used once, more than once or not at all.

Lead-in: For each of the following patients with formal thought disorder, choose the term above that best fits what is described.

Stems:

85.1   A 31-year-old man was asked about his appetite. He replied, 'I never have trouble eating. I never have trouble peeping. I never have trouble beeping.'

85.2   The symptom he has exhibited is common in which of the above disorders?

85.3   A 40-year-old woman was asked about whether she had trouble sleeping during the night. She replied, 'I used to sleep in my bed but now I'm sleeping on the sofa.'

85.4   A 17-year-old girl described her daily routine activities as follows: 'I ... I watch TV, dad does not come home, I ... mother is at home too. Sometimes, its better to rain, you know. Betty smokes a lot.'

Question 86. *Psychopathological features occasionally seen in schizophrenia.*

Theme: Psychopathological features occasionally seen in schizophrenia.

Options:

A.	Advertence.	F.	*Flexibilitas cerea.*
B.	Age disorientation.	G.	Metonymy.
C.	Clang association.	H.	Neologism.
D.	Cryptolalia.	I.	Psychological pillow.
E.	*Doppelgänger* phenomenon.	J.	*Schnauzkrampf.*

Each option may be used once, more than once or not at all.

Lead-in: Choose the psychopathology term above that most closely describes what each of the following patients with schizophrenia is experiencing.

Stems:

86.1 A man is convinced that he has seen himself on a number of occasions while walking about in his local town. He knows that this sighting was of himself as he feels an awareness of himself both inside and outside his body. He fears that this bodes ill for the future.

86.2 A 55-year-old woman who has been a backward inpatient for thirty years says '48' when asked her age.

86.3 A man is noted to lie for hours on his ward bed with his head raised three inches off the bed.

86.4 A woman speaks rapidly in a language that no one can make out. Collateral history from her family reveals that she did not do any languages at school.

Question 87. Panic disorder

Theme: Panic disorder.

Options: A.   A few minutes.
                B.   A few seconds.
                C.   Anticipatory fear.
                D.   Dependency.
                E.   Dramatising.
                F.   Hours.
                G.   Non-situational and expected.
                H.   Non-situational and unexpected.
                I.   Occasional secondary fear.
                J.   Secondary fear is almost invariable.
                K.   Secondary fear is common.
                L.   Situational and unexpected.

Each option may be used once, more than once or not at all.

Lead-in: A 30-year-old housewife has a two-year history of
                unpredictable recurrent attacks of severe anxiety that are
                not restricted to any particular situation or circumstances.
                For each of the following questions, select the most
                appropriate answer above.

Stems: 87.1   She has become reluctant to be alone in public
                       places away from home. She has developed this
                       symptom due to which psychological mechanism?

              87.2   How is the occurrence of typical panic attacks best
                       described?

              87.3   Her typical individual attacks will commonly last
                       for what duration?

              87.4   Secondary fear of dying, losing control or going mad
                       occurs at what frequency in panic disorder?

Question 88. First-rank symptoms of schizophrenia

Theme: First-rank symptoms of schizophrenia.

Options: A.   Arguing third person voices.
             B.   Audible thoughts.
             C.   Commenting third person voices.
             D.   Delusional perception.
             E.   Made action.
             F.   Made feeling.
             G.   Made impulse.
             H.   Somatic passivity.
             I.   Thought broadcasting.
             J.   Thought insertion.
             K.   Thought withdrawal.

Each option may be used once, more than once or not at all.

Lead-in: Select the first-rank symptom of schizophrenia above that
             most closely describes what the following patients have
             been experiencing.

Stems: 88.1   'When I saw that my neighbour had left the door of
                    his tractor open, I realised that I was destined to be
                    the High Commissioner of the European Union. I
                    wrote to them to say I was ready but have not got a
                    reply yet: I fear Al-Qaeda are blocking my
                    appointment.'

             88.2   'The IRA has a device that can tap into mobile phone
                    transmitters. They are using it to create an urge in
                    me to defecate no matter where I am. When they do
                    this, I usually decide to do what they want.'

             88.3   'The First Minister of the Welsh Parliament has been
                    broadcasting party political briefings into my head
                    and is trying to swamp my thoughts with his quasi-
                    geopolitical ranting.'

             88.4   'The England soccer team are using a hypnotherapist
                    to hinder me when I play football. Whenever I am in
                    a position to score she sends thoughts that cause pain
                    and weakness in my right leg that cause me to miss.'

Question 89. Psychopathological terms from German psychiatry

Theme: Psychopathological terms from German psychiatry.

Options: A.   *Doppelgänger.*   F.   *Schnauzkrampf.*
               B.   *Gedankenlautwerden.*   G.   *Verstimmung.*
               C.   *Gegenhalten.*   H.   *Vorbeigehen.*
               D.   *Mitgehen.*   I.   *Wahnstimmung.*
               E.   *Mitmachen.*   J.   *Witzelsucht.*

Each option may be used once, more than once or not at all.

Lead-in: From the following descriptions, choose the most
               appropriate term above that refers to the phenomenon.

Stems: 89.1 A 21-year-old female reports being distressed by
                     the experience of having her thoughts spoken aloud
                     behind her in a low whisper at the same time that
                     she thinks them.

               89.2 A 27-year-old male is propelled across the room by
                     a tiny push from the tip of the examiner's index
                     finger despite being told to resist any attempts at
                     moving him.

               89.3 A 56-year-old man is noted to have a peculiar
                     grimace: his nose and lips are protruded forward
                     and make as if to meet each other.

               89.4 A 33-year-old woman is perplexed and
                     apprehensive, feeling something of great importance
                     is about to occur connected with her, but is unable
                     to tell what this will be.

Question 90. Speech disorders

Theme: Speech disorders.

Options: A.   Circumstantiality.
               B.   Derailment.
               C.   Echolalia.
               D.   Fusion.
               E.   Jargon aphasia.
               F.   Logoclonia.
               G.   Palilalia.
               H.   Paraphasia.
               I.   Verbigeration.
               J.   *Vorbeigehen.*

Each option may be used once only or not at all.

Lead-in: For each of the following conversations, select the term
               above that describes the patient's speech disorder most
               closely.

Stems: 90.1   **Examiner:** 'How many legs do ducks have?'
                      Subject: 'Three'
                      Examiner: 'What colour is the sky?'
                      Subject: 'Pink'

               90.2   **Examiner:** 'What brought you here today?'
                      Subject: 'I was coming to the room but there was
                      no brush. I saw it was windy with my head in my
                      hands.'

               90.3   **Examiner:** 'How are you feeling today?'
                      Subject: '... I still have the same sadness-ness-
                      ness.'
                      Examiner: 'Is your mood any better than
                      yesterday?'
                      Subject: '... No, I still feel terrible-ble-ble.'

Question 91. Sensory distortions

Theme: Sensory distortions.

Options: A.   Chloropsia.   F.   Micropsia.
              B.   Dysmegalopsia.   G.   Porropsia.
              C.   Hyperacusis.   H.   Splitting of perception.
              D.   Hypoacusis.   I.   Visual hyperaesthesia.
              E.   Macropsia.   J.   Visual hypoaesthesia.

Each option may be used once, more than once or not at all.

Lead-in: For each of the following individuals with sensory
              distortions, choose the term above that most closely
              describes his/her experience.

Stems: 91.1   A 54-year-old man with alcohol dependence is
                     being treated for delirium tremens in hospital. He
                     does not respond to the member of the domestic
                     staff when she asks him what he wants for dinner
                     until she raises her voice considerably.

              91.2   An 18-year-old woman with epilepsy often notices
                     objects to be larger on one side than the other when
                     a seizure is about to commence.

              91.3   A 48-year-old woman with depression no longer
                     enjoys her flower garden. She states that their
                     former brilliant colours seem to have faded, and all
                     now seem dull.

              91.4   A 73-year-old man with no psychiatric history sees
                     a car driving towards him. He can see the car
                     clearly and hears its engine, but experiences the
                     two sensations as being separate, unrelated
                     occurrences.

Question 92. Hallucinatory experiences

Theme: Hallucinatory experiences.

Options: A.   Autoscopic hallucination.
               B.   Elementary hallucination.
               C.   Extracampine hallucination.
               D.   Functional hallucination.
               E.   Hygric hallucination.
               F.   Hypnagogic hallucination.
               G.   Hypnopompic hallucination.
               H.   Kinaesthetic hallucination.
               I.   Lilliputian hallucination.
               J.   Negative autoscopic hallucination.
               K.   Reduplicative hallucination.
               L.   Reflex hallucination.

Each option may be used once, more than once or not at all.

Lead-in: For each of the following vignettes, choose the term above
               that most closely describes the hallucinatory experience.

Stems: 92.1   A 75-year-old woman cries when see looks into the
                      mirror to see that she has no reflection.

               92.2   A 22-year-old man stabs himself to try to release
                      the fluid he feels gradually filling up and
                      overflowing from his abdomen into his chest.

               92.3   A 34-year-old man experiences severe numbness in
                      his right leg whenever the radio is switched on.

               92.4   A 55-year-old woman asks her general practitioner
                      to arrange for the amputation of a third upper limb
                      that she feels she has developed.

Question 93. *Disorders of mood and affect*

Theme: Disorders of mood and affect.

Options: A.   Alexithymia.   F.   Ecstasy.
               B.   Anhedonia.   G.   Elation.
               C.   Apathy.   H.   Euphoria.
               D.   Blunted affect.   I.   Flattened affect.
               E.   Depression.   J.   Labile affect.

Each option may be used once, more than once or not at all.

Lead-in: For each of the following patients, choose the term above
               that most closely describes his or her mood/affect state.

Stems: 93.1   A 25-year-old woman with schizophrenia is
                      observed over time by the hostel staff. She does not
                      seem to display much emotion, and when she does
                      it is less than one would expect but it is usually
                      appropriate to the situation.

               93.2   A 64-year-old man with schizophrenia appears to
                      have no emotional reactions whatsoever. When this
                      is put to him by his doctor, he considers it and
                      agrees that this has been the case for quite some
                      time.

               93.3   A 30-year-old man has great difficulty in expressing
                      how he is feeling. He also reports, when questioned,
                      having few daydreams and infrequent dreams at
                      night.

               93.4   A 55-year-old woman attends a special Catholic
                      service to which the relics of a venerated saint are
                      brought by a visiting cardinal. She describes a
                      moment of sublime happiness during the service,
                      during which she felt 'as if I was at one with God's
                      plan'.

Question 94. Psychopathological features of delirium

Theme: Psychopathological features of delirium.

Options: A.   Affect illusion.
            B.   Concrete thinking.
            C.   Delusion of persecution.
            D.   Elementary hallucination.
            E.   Ideas of reference.
            F.   Impoverished thought.
            G.   Hypoacusis.
            H.   Lilliputian hallucinations.
            I.   Occupational delirium.
            J.   Pareidolia.
            K.   Perseveration.
            L.   Reduplicative paramnesia.

Each option may be used once, more than once or not at all.

Lead-in: For each of following patients with an acute organic
            reaction, choose the descriptive psychopathological term
            above that most closely describes what is occurring.

Stems: 94.1   A dehydrated elderly woman sits quietly in her bed
                looking terrified. When the nurses wheel in the drug
                trolley, she screams aloud as she perceives it as a
                coffin they are pushing.

            94.2   An elderly farmer who is taking a number of drugs
                with anticholinergic activity sits up late at night
                because he is convinced there are people who are
                determined to steal his cows.

            94.3   A middle-aged man with raised intracranial pressure
                is asked to explain the proverb 'far-away hills are
                greener'. He replies that this is because there are
                probably better fields there.

            94.4   A retired teacher with a lower respiratory tract
                infection believes that the hospital is her old school
                and can point out the various 'classrooms', which
                are in fact the various wards in the hospital.

Question 95. Delusional disorder

Theme: Delusional disorder.

Options: A.   Autoscopy.
B.   Capgras' syndrome.
C.   Cotard's syndrome.
D.   De Clérambault's syndrome.
E.   Delusional jealously.
F.   Fregoli delusion.
G.   *Illusion de sosies.*
H.   Intermetamorphosis delusion.
I.   Reverse subjective double syndrome.
J.   Subjective doubles delusion.

Each option may be used once, more than once or not at all.

Lead-in: For each of the following patients with delusional beliefs, choose the term above that most closely describes what they are experiencing.

Stems: 95.1   A man believes that he can see others temporarily changing into someone else in both external appearance and personality.

95.2   A young woman believes that her double exists and is functioning independently.

95.3   A woman thinks that she is being replaced psychologically by someone else.

95.4   A young woman has followed a pop star on tour for three years, believing that he is in love with her. She has made threats to kill his children if he does not publicly admit his love for her.

Question 96. Psychodynamic theorists

Theme: Psychodynamic theorists.

Options: A. Actual self.   G. Masculine protest.
                B. Animus.   H. Psychobiology.
                C. Holistic approach.   I. Pathological mother.
                D. Idealized self.   J. Shadow.
                E. Individual psychology.   K. Synchronicity.
                F. Inferiority complex.   L. Transitional object.

Each option may be once only.

Lead-in: For each of the following psychodynamic theorists, select
                the required number of concepts above that are most
                associated with that theorist.

Stems: 96.1   Alfred Adler. *(Choose three items)*

                96.2   Carl Gustav Jung. *(Choose three items)*

                96.3   Adolf Meyer. *(Choose two items)*

                96.4   Donald Winnicott. *(Choose two items)*

Question 97. Depersonalisation and derealisation

Theme: Depersonalisation and derealisation.

Options: A.   Emotional apathy.
B.   Familiarity of unfamiliar objects.
C.   Familiarity of unfamiliar person.
D.   Incongruous emotions.
E.   Localisation of depersonalisation to an individual organ.
F.   Loss of capacity to feel emotions.
G.   Loss of capacity to feel normal sensations.
H.   Loss of capacity to feel sensory symptoms of organic illness.
I.   Unfamiliarity of familiar objects.
J.   Unfamiliarity of familiar person.

Each option may be used once, more than once or not at all.

Lead-in: Abnormal personal experiences with awareness are known by different terms. Choose the definition above that best fits each of the following terms.

Stems: 97.1   De-affectualisation.

97.2   De-somatisation.

97.3   *Déjà vu.*

97.4   *Jamais vu.*

Question 98. Generalised anxiety disorder

Theme: Generalised anxiety disorder.

Options: A.   Autonomic hyperresponsiveness.
                B.   Autonomic hyporesponsiveness.
                C.   Fear.
                D.   Increased prevalence of past trauma.
                E.   Obsessive rumination.
                F.   One year.
                G.   Six months.
                H.   Three months.
                I.   Unresolved oedipal conflict.
                J.   Worry.

Each option may be used once, more than once or not at all.

Lead-in: A young male has a history of generalised anxiety disorder
                based on an ICD-10 diagnosis instrument. Choose the
                phrase above that best answers each of the following
                questions about him.

Stems: 98.1   He has a chain of thoughts that have a negative
                       affective content concerned with future events
                       where there is uncertainty of outcome. This feature
                       is known as what?

                98.2   He is likely to show which autonomic response to a
                       stress challenge?

                98.3   Which of the above features, according to
                       psychodynamic theory, is he most likely to have?

                98.4   What is the minimum period of time that
                       symptoms must be present to diagnose generalised
                       anxiety disorder using ICD-10?

Question 99. *Paranoid schizophrenia*

Theme: Paranoid schizophrenia.

Options: A.   Autochthonus delusion.
B.   Autonomy *versus* shame and doubt.
C.   Denial and projection.
D.   First-rank symptom.
E.   Industry *versus* inferiority.
F.   Introjection and projection.
G.   Reaction formation and projection.
H.   Second-rank symptom.
I.   Secondary delusion.
J.   Trust *versus* mistrust.

Each option may be used once, more than once or not at all.

Lead-in: A 40-year-old-man is convinced that the IRA is spying on him and trying to kill him. He is certain that there were two men with hidden guns who visited the hospital ward yesterday to shoot him. He came to this conclusion as he heard multiple voices plotting to kill him.

Answer each of the following questions with the phrase above that most closely fits what he is experiencing.

Stems: 99.1   To which of Kurt Schneider's rankings does his hallucination belong?

99.2   To which of Kurt Schneider's rankings does his delusional beliefs belong?

99.3   According to Freud, what are the defence mechanisms responsible for his delusions?

99.4   Which psychosocial stage of Erikson is associated with paranoid thoughts?

Question 100. Pioneers of psychodynamic theory

Theme: Pioneers of psychodynamic theory.

Options: A.   Alfred Adler.
              B.   Anna Freud.
              C.   Carl Jung.
              D.   Eric Berne.
              E.   Erik Erikson.
              F.   Harry Stack Sullivan.
              G.   Melanie Klein.
              H.   Otto Kernberg.
              I.   Otto Rank.
              J.   Wilhelm Reich.

Each option may be used once only or not at all.

Lead-in: For each of the following individual brief descriptions of
              psychodynamic theory, choose the theorist above most
              closely associated with its development.

Stems: 100.1   Neurosis comes from sexual energy, the release of
                      which has been blocked. These tensions form
                      physical tensions that reflect the underlying
                      character armour of the individual. Therapy
                      involves analysing this prior to attempting to
                      analyse the unconscious.

              100.2   All neuroses do not come from repressed libidinal
                      desires. Individuals are future-directed by nature,
                      and so choose life-goals shaped by their
                      interpersonal environment. Inappropriate goals
                      can lead to neurosis. Psychosis results from the
                      individual losing social interest and retreating into
                      himself.

              100.3   Individuals develop through a series of stages of
                      cognitive and social development as children.
                      Excessive anxiety interferes with the development
                      of the self-system and can cause an arrest in
                      development at a particular stage. Transference, or
                      parataxic distortions, may occur in all human
                      interactions, not just the psychoanalytical
                      relationship.

Question 101. Delusions

Theme: Delusions.

Options: A.   Both primary and secondary delusions.
                 B.   Delusional memory.
                 C.   Delusional mood.
                 D.   Delusional percept.
                 E.   Primary delusions.
                 F.   Secondary delusions.

Each option may be used once, more than once or not at all.

Lead-in: Delusions can be classified based on the characteristics of their contents. Choose the phrase above that best answers the following questions on each of these patients' delusions.

Stems: 101.1   A middle-aged man who has a history of impotence claims that strangers jump into his house through the roof at nighttime, hypnotise him and then interfere with him sexually. He also believes that his employer is using satellite connections to observe him.

                         Of which broad category of delusions are these delusions an example?

                 101.2   A middle-aged Buddhist woman believed that her neighbours would not accept her religious beliefs and felt that they might be hostile, but she could not define quite how. She kept checking that her neighbours could not hear what she was saying in her home and appeared anxious and puzzled.

                         Which term best describes her experience?

Question 102. *Auditory hallucinations*

Theme: Auditory hallucinations.

Options: A.   Arguing voices.
                B.   Command hallucination.
                C.   *Écho de pensée.*
                D.   Elementary hallucination.
                E.   *Gedankenlautwerden.*
                F.   Running commentary.
                G.   Second person hallucination.
                H.   Third person hallucination.

Each option may be used once, more than once or not at all.

Lead-in: Each of the following descriptions is an auditory
                hallucination heard by a patient. Choose all of the
                appropriate items above that describe what is being
                experienced.

Stems: 102.1   'Look at what she's doing now, she's tidying up
                         her breakfast dishes and putting them into the
                         sink. Now she's leaving them unwashed as she
                         goes to collect her handbag.'

                102.2   **Male voice:** 'Look at what the useless sod *[i.e. the
                         patient]* is wearing!'
                         Female voice: 'Shut up, leave him alone, he's all
                         right.'
                         Male voice: 'Don't tell me to shut up, I've more
                         right to be here than you.'

                102.3   'Oh hell, I'm running late…no time for breakfast,
                         I'll grab a quick coffee when I get to work…where
                         did I leave my car keys?'
                         *[These are the exact thoughts of the patient, spoken
                         aloud behind her at the same time she thinks them.]*

                102.4   'Uh-Uh-Uh-Wheeeee-Ssssssssh.'

Question 103. Delirium

Theme: Delirium.

Options:
A. Automatism.
B. Coma.
C. Delirium tremens.
D. Drowsiness
E. *Mania à potu.*
F. Oneiroid state.
G. Stupor.
H. Twilight state.

Each option may be used once, more than once or not at all.

Lead-in: For each of the following patients with altered states of consciousness, choose the condition above that is most likely to be responsible for his/her behaviour.

Stems:
103.1 A 45-year-old man acutely developed tachycardia, sweating, coarse tremor, dehydration and raised temperature associated with seeing little men shouting obscene jokes and abusive remarks in his ear.

103.2 A 30-year-old man acutely developed an inappropriate, complex, coordinated, purposeful and directed involuntary behaviour for which he had only partial memory.

103.3 A 28-year-old man abruptly and unexpectedly displayed violence that lasted for three hours.

Question 104. Disorders of consciousness

Theme: Disorders of consciousness.

Options: A.   Akinetic mutism.
              B.   Automatism.
              C.   Clouding of consciousness.
              D.   Drowsiness.
              E.   Locked-in syndrome.
              F.   *Mania à potu.*
              G.   Oneiroid state.
              H.   Twilight state.

Each option may be used once, more than once or not at all.

Lead-in: Each of the following patients has a disorder of
              consciousness. Choose the term above that most closely
              describes his/her state.

Stems: 104.1   A 56-year-old man is awake on the ward, but
                       drifts off to sleep unless there is some activity
                       going on near him. When questioned, he answers
                       slowly and has slurred speech. His muscle tone is
                       reduced on examination.

              104.2   A 72-year-old former tailor is markedly confused
                       in his nursing home, and is making a nuisance of
                       himself going to each individual and 'measuring'
                       them for a new suit with a piece of string he has
                       found.

              104.3   A 32-year-old woman with temporal lobe epilepsy
                       has had a number of episodes that occur all of a
                       sudden and last for about three hours, in which
                       she is uncharacteristically hostile, and she has hit
                       her husband severely on occasion during these
                       spells.

              104.4   A 22-year-old woman has two glasses of wine
                       with her boyfriend and abruptly tries to attack
                       him with the bottle, despite this being highly
                       uncharacteristic behaviour for her. Following the
                       episode, she sleeps for 20 hours and states she
                       remembers little of the event when she wakes up.

Question 105. Perceptual disorder

Theme: Perceptual disorder.

Options: A.   First person.
              B.   Hallucinemes.
              C.   Morphemes.
              D.   Peremptory orders.
              E.   Phonemes.
              F.   Running commentary.
              G.   Second person.
              H.   Short, abusive remarks.
              I.   Third person.
              J.   Unstructured sounds.

Each option may be used once only.

Lead-in: A 25-year-old man states that he can hear voices when
              there is nobody around. Answer each of the following
              questions with the most appropriate phrase or phrases
              above.

Stems: 105.1   What characteristics of hallucinations above
                      would most support a diagnosis of schizophrenia?
                      (Select two options)

              105.2   In which person would the voices be most likely
                      to occur, if there were an organic cause for his
                      hallucinations? (Select one option)

              105.3   What term is sometimes used to denote such
                      voices? (Select one option)

Question 106. *Alcoholism and cognitive impairment*

Theme: Alcoholism and cognitive impairment.

Options: A.   Alcoholic dementia.
                B.   Confabulation of embarrassment.
                C.   Dissociative amnesia.
                D.   Echolalia.
                E.   Fantastic confabulation.
                F.   Ganser syndrome.
                G.   Korsakoff psychosis.
                H.   Mamillary body.
                I.   Negativism.
                J.   Parietal lobe.
                K.   Subthalamic nucleus.
                L.   Suggestibility.

Each option may be used once only.

Lead-in: A 45-year-old man tries to cover up an exposed memory
                gap with false information. He has a long history of
                alcoholism. When the therapist prompted different
                information, the patient readily changed his statement
                even though this was contradicting what he said
                previously. He does not attempt to correct these
                inconsistencies.

                *Choose the term above that best answers each of the following
                questions about this man's condition.*

Stems: 106.1   What is his most likely diagnosis?

                106.2   What term above best describes his offering of
                        false information to the interviewer?

                106.3   What characteristic is being displayed when the
                        patient changes his story in response to the
                        therapist offering different information?

                106.4   Lesions of which part of the brain are associated
                        with this clinical presentation?

Question 107. Methods of controlling thoughts and impulses

Theme:　　Methods of controlling thoughts and impulses.

Options:　A.　Blocking.
　　　　　　B.　Controlling.
　　　　　　C.　Denial.
　　　　　　D.　Inhibition.
　　　　　　E.　Isolation.
　　　　　　F.　Primary repression.
　　　　　　G.　Regression.
　　　　　　H.　Secondary repression.
　　　　　　I.　Sublimation.
　　　　　　J.　Suppression.

Each option may be used once, more than once or not at all.

Lead-in:　Which of the above defence mechanisms best explains the following behaviour?

Stems:　　107.1　A 17-year-old man becomes tense when he inhibits his thoughts of harming his father from his conscious awareness for the time being.

　　　　　　107.2　A 25-year-old married man postpones his wish to confront his wife when she told him a lie for the time being.

　　　　　　107.3　A 16-year-old girl withholds the sexual feelings she once experienced towards her father from her conscious perception.

　　　　　　107.4　A 35-year-old mother continues to be anxious even after successfully expelling her thoughts to kill her child from conscious perception.

Question 108. Object relations

Theme: Object relations.

Options: A.   Antilibidinal object.
                B.   Depressive position.
                C.   Dissociation.
                D.   Ideal object.
                E.   Libidinal object.
                F.   Paranoid-schizoid position.
                G.   Projective identification.
                H.   Reaction formation.
                I.   The good, but not perfect, mother.
                J.   The perfect mother who is always in tune with her
                      infant's needs.

Each option may be used once, more than once or not at all.

Lead-in: Choose the concept of object relations theory above that
                best answers each of the following questions.

Stems: 108.1   Winnicott felt that the development of the infant
                       would best be helped by having a mother with
                       which characteristics?

              108.2   According to Fairburn, the object that could
                       satisfy the child's drive-related needs is known as
                       what object?

              108.3   According to Klein the child develops integration,
                       responsibility and concern for the object in which
                       development position?

              108.4   When one member of a couple has an affair and
                       the hurt member of the couple retaliates by
                       sleeping with someone else, this is an example of
                       which defence mechanism?

Question 109. Psychodynamics of depression

Theme: Psychodynamics of depression.

Options: A.   Ambivalency.
               B.   Automatic thoughts.
               C.   Internally-directed anger.
               D.   Projective-identification.
               E.   Rationalisation.
               F.   Reaction formation.
               G.   Reactivation of depressive position.
               H.   Reactivation of paranoid position.
               I.   Regression.
               J.   Sublimation.

Each option may be used once, more than once or not at all.

Lead-in: A 36-year-old woman has been feeling sad, irritable and
               angry for the last three weeks. She feels guilty to be a
               burden on her family. She also regrets not being with her
               father when he died several years ago. She believes that
               she deserves punishment and to rot in hell because of
               these perceived wrongdoings.

               *For each of the following questions, choose the mechanism above
               that is most likely to be implicated.*

Stems: 109.1   Freud understood these feelings as a harsh
                       superego that punishes the person for harbouring
                       destructive wishes towards parental figures. What
                       mechanism did he suggest is responsible for this?

               109.2   Melanie Klein suggested that depressed patients
                       are convinced that they have destroyed their
                       internal good objects because of their own
                       aggression; they feel persecuted by internal bad
                       objects. What is the mechanism involved here
                       known as?

Clinical Theory and Skills
EMIs

Question 110. *Conducting the psychiatric interview*

Theme: Conducting the psychiatric interview.

Options: A.   Ask for a chaperone.
B.   Check what the patient means.
C.   Ensure escape is possible.
D.   Pretend to empathise.
E.   React to her emotion.
F.   Refrain from making notes.
G.   Speak with a loud tone.
H.   Stroke her knee.
I.   Use closed questions.
J.   Use her first name.

Each option may be used once, more than once or not at all.

Lead-in: Each of the following depicts a different situation in which you have to interview a 26-year-old female who has presented as an emergency psychiatric referral. *Based on the information that you have just been given in each stem*, choose the most salient action above as to how you would act.

Stems: 110.1   The patient tells you that she is very 'paranoid' at the moment.

110.2   When you call the patient into the interview room, you address her as 'Ms Fox'. She asks you to call her by her first name instead.

110.3   Soon after beginning the interview, she breaks into tears unexpectedly.

110.4   While the room has an adequate layout and alarm system, upon showing the patient to the interview room you are concerned to note a marked flirtatiousness in her demeanour combined with a provocative manner of dress.

Question 111. ICD-10 diagnoses

Theme: ICD-10 diagnoses.

Options: A.   Adjustment disorder.
                   B.   Brief recurrent depressive disorder.
                   C.   Cyclothymia.
                   D.   Dysthymia.
                   E.   Moderate depressive episode.
                   F.   Recurrent depressive disorder.
                   G.   Seasonal affective disorder.
                   H.   Severe depressive episode without psychotic symptoms.
                   I.   Severe depressive episode with psychotic symptoms.

Each option may be used once, more than once or not at all.

Lead-in: Choose the ICD-10 diagnosis above that most closely fits each of the case summaries given below.

Stems: 111.1   Following a business partner's death three months ago, a 55-year-old self-employed businessman developed the following symptoms: inability to work, poor concentration, disturbed sleep, poor appetite, loss of sexual interest, and decreased energy. He became convinced that he was already bankrupt. He developed all of these symptoms in the last three weeks.

                  111.2   A 36-year-old housewife has a history of short transient moderate depressive episodes lasting for four or five days, occurring several times in a year for no apparent reason.

                  111.3   A 28-year-old male bank employee has an eight-year history of low mood, lethargy, feelings of laziness, and decreased energy. He states his mood is worse in the evenings, and has negative feelings about himself and his future. These symptoms last for several months at a time and he reports times of feeling normal in between episodes that generally last for a few days.

Question 112. Concepts of schizophrenia

Theme: Concepts of schizophrenia.

Options: A.   Anhedonia.
                B.   Autism.
                C.   Autoscopy.
                D.   Biological.
                E.   One.
                F.   Psychobiological.
                G.   Psychological.
                H.   Psychosocial.
                I.   Three.
                J.   Two.

Each option may be used once, more than once or not at all.

Lead-in: A 30-year-old female has a three-year history of hearing
                her own thoughts spoken aloud, thinking that her uterus is
                missing since she has been gang raped two years ago,
                repeating others' gestures, talking very slowly and
                inaudibly, and being emotionally apathetic.

                *Choose the option above that most closely answers each of the
                following questions.*

Stems: 112.1   Which of the above did Bleuler regard as one of
                         the fundamental features of this disorder?

                112.2   How many of Kurt Schneider's first-rank
                         symptoms does she exhibit?

                112.3   Which mechanism did Kraepelin describe as the
                         main aetiological factor for her disorder?

                112.4   Which mechanism did Bleuler believe was the
                         main aetiological factor for her disorder?

Question 113. *Clinical progression of dementias*

Theme: Clinical progression of dementias.

Options: A.   Dementia in Creutzfeldt-Jakob disease.
               B.   Dementia in HIV disease.
               C.   Dementia in Huntington's disease.
               D.   Dementia in general paralysis of the insane.
               E.   Dementia in Parkinson's disease.
               F.   Multi-infarct dementia.
               G.   Pick's disease.
               H.   Post-encephalitic parkinsonism.
               I.   Pseudo-bulbar palsy.

Each option may be used once, more than once or not at all.

Lead-in: For each of the clinical scenarios of dementia described
               below choose the most likely diagnosis above.

Stems: 113.1   A 50-year-old man has developed rapidly
                       progressing dementia for the last thirteen months,
                       which is associated with Parkinsonian tremor and
                       rigidity, myoclonus and triphasic waves on the
                       electroencephalogram.

               113.2   A 55-year-old woman has a slow progressive
                       dementia of nine years' duration, with choreiform
                       movements of the face and hands, and has an
                       abnormal gait. There is a positive family history of
                       similar disease.

               113.3   A 60-year-old man has a history of impaired
                       cognitive functions that are unevenly impaired,
                       associated with a history of hypertension,
                       emotional lability, and transient episodes of
                       delirium. His insight into his condition is
                       preserved.

Question 114. Interviewing the patient

Theme: Interviewing the patient.

Options: A.   Depressed patients.
               B.   Highly suspicious patients.
               C.   Patients who lie.
               D.   Patients with thought-block.
               E.   Potentially violent patients.
               F.   Seductive patients.

Each option may be used once, more than once or not at all.

Lead-in: Interview strategies for different groups of patients are
               described below. Choose the type of patients above for
               whom each strategy is *most* intended.

Stems: 114.1   Efforts to reassure or ingratiate should be avoided
                       in these patients.

               114.2   A more forceful and directive technique than
                       usual may be helpful in the evaluation of these
                       patients.

               114.3   For these patients, the interview should be
                       conducted in a quiet, non-stimulating
                       environment.

               114.4   With this group of patients, a respectful insistence
                       that the previously-negotiated form of payment
                       for treatment be adhered to may be necessary.

Question 115. Schizophrenia

Theme: Schizophrenia.

Options: A.   Catatonic schizophrenia.
B.   Hebephrenic schizophrenia.
C.   Paranoid schizophrenia.
D.   Persistent delusional disorder.
E.   Post-schizophrenic depression.
F.   Residual schizophrenia.
G.   Schizotypal disorder.
H.   Schizoaffective disorder, depressive type.
I.   Undifferentiated schizophrenia.

Each option may be used once, more than once or not at all.

Lead-in: For each of the following patients with a psychotic disorder, choose the ICD-10 diagnosis above that best fits the clinical picture.

Stems: 115.1   An 18-year-old boy has a nine-month history of shallow affect, mannerisms, multiple somatic complaints and incoherent speech. He is withdrawn and describes hearing multiple voices telling him different kinds of information.

115.2   A 40-year-old woman has been on treatment for schizophrenia with an atypical antipsychotic for the last seven months. Her delusions and hallucinations remain prominent despite the antipsychotic treatment. She also has depressed mood, feelings of hopelessness, and decreased energy and appetite for the last seven days.

115.3   A 24-year-old male has a six-month history of talking and laughing to himself. He hears voices talking to him critically and neglects his personal hygiene. He is uncommunicative most of the time. He has also damaged property and assaulted strangers for no apparent reason. Often, he assumes uncomfortable postures for hours for no obvious reason.

Question 116. Dementia

Theme: Dementia.

Options:
- A. AIDS dementia.
- B. Alcoholic dementia.
- C. Alzheimer's disease.
- D. Dementia associated with Parkinson's disease.
- E. Dementia of Lewy body type.
- F. Huntington's disease.
- G. Pick's disease.
- H. Vascular dementia.
- I. Wilson's disease.

Each option may be used once, more than once or not at all.

Lead-in: A 65-year-old man had progressive multiple cognitive deficits, memory impairment, difficulties in executive functioning and personality deterioration before his death.

For each of the following separate scenarios of autopsy and histopathological findings, select from the list above the dementia above most likely to be responsible for his symptoms:

Stems: 116.1 The autopsy revealed widened sulci in the temporal, parietal and frontal lobes. There were extensive senile plaques in the hippocampus and neo-cortex, with neurofibrillary tangles, and cholinergic neuronal loss in the nucleus of Meynert.

116.2 The brain had extensive Lewy bodies in the temporal lobe, cingulate gyrus and insular cortex. There was moderate loss of nigral dopaminergic neurons, together with a few senile plaques and neurofibrillary tangles.

116.3 Neuronal loss was prominent in the frontal lobes, and striatum. There was atrophy of the head of caudate and putamen. Loss of striatal GABAergic neurons was seen and there was increased dopaminergic concentration in the basal ganglia.

Question 117. Anxiety disorders in DSM-IV

Theme: Anxiety disorders in DSM-IV.

Options: A.   Acute stress disorder.
                B.   Agoraphobia.
                C.   Anxiety disorder not otherwise specified.
                D.   Generalized anxiety disorder.
                E.   Obsessive-compulsive disorder.
                F.   Panic disorder.
                G.   Post-traumatic stress disorder.
                H.   Social phobia.
                I.   Specific phobia.
                J.   Substance-induced anxiety disorder.

Each option may be used once, more than once or not at all.

Lead-in: For each of the following patients with anxiety symptoms,
                select the most likely diagnosis above.

Stems: 117.1   A 29-year-old woman from Edinburgh can only
                        leave her house in the company of her husband, as
                        she fears having further panic attacks. She refuses
                        to travel in any vehicle except a car in case she
                        needs to get out quickly should she panic. Her
                        panic attacks also occur unexpectedly in situations
                        such as watching television or doing housework.

                117.2   A 45-year-old man from Dublin with newly
                        diagnosed haemochromatosis is finding difficulties
                        with the monitoring and treatment of his condition,
                        as he tends to faint whenever he sees blood or has
                        to have an injection.

                117.3   A 60-year-old woman from Birmingham has to
                        check the gas is off and all the doors are locked at
                        night ten times each, while repeating 'nothing will
                        happen on my watch', otherwise she will worry
                        about them. This takes about twenty minutes to
                        perform each night and she admits feeling slightly
                        distressed by this.

                117.4   A 31-year-old man from Tokyo tends to avoid
                        meeting people where possible, as he fears that his
                        eye contact and body odours will give offence to
                        others. Otherwise, he denies particular feelings of
                        embarrassment in social situations and realises his
                        concerns are excessive.

Question 118. Anorexia nervosa

Theme: Anorexia nervosa.

Options:
    A. Delayed gastric emptying.
    B. Does not gauge the size of other people correctly.
    C. Gauges her own size correctly.
    D. Gauges the size of inanimate objects correctly.
    E. Hypervitaminosis.
    F. Normal vitamin levels.
    G. Rapid gastric emptying.
    H. To make herself more attractive to others.
    I. To satisfy herself.
    J. Vitamin deficiencies.

Each option may be used once, more than once or not at all.

Lead-in: A 5′6″ 18-year-old woman weighs 5 stone 6 pounds. She eats a sandwich every day in the evening and drinks plenty of water and diet orange juice. She would prefer to weigh less than 5 stone and she finds her body bulky and unattractive.

Answer each of the following questions about her, using the most appropriate phrase above.

Stems:
    118.1 Typically, what does she want to achieve by losing this weight?

    118.2 How is her ability to gauge size best described?

    118.3 What is her most likely vitamin profile?

    118.4 How is her gastric emptying likely to be affected?

Question 119. Social causation of schizophrenia

Theme: Social causation of schizophrenia.

Options: A.   Abnormal family communication.
                B.   Breeder hypothesis.
                C.   Double-bind.
                D.   Drifter hypothesis.
                E.   Emotional overinvolvement.
                F.   Expressed emotion.
                G.   Marital skew.
                H.   Marital schism.
                I.   Mortification process.
                J.   Schizophrenogenic mother.

Each option may be used once, more than once or not at all.

Lead-in: Select the most appropriate terms above that describe the
                sociological theories of the aetiology/risk factor of
                schizophrenia described below.

Stems: 119.1   The child of an eccentric mother who is the more
                         powerful in the marriage, the father remaining
                         passive, will have an increased risk of later
                         schizophrenia.

                119.2   A mother constantly gives mixed messages to her
                         son such as telling him she loves him while glaring
                         ferociously at him. This puts the child at an
                         increased risk of later schizophrenia.

                119.3   A mother has a number of characteristics such as
                         indifference, hostility and overprotectiveness
                         towards her child, thereby putting him at
                         increased risk of schizophrenia.

                119.4   The deprivation experience by those from lower
                         socio-economic groups, particularly those in urban
                         areas, is a direct causative factor for
                         schizophrenia.

Question 120. Clinical manifestations of somatoform disorders

Theme: Clinical manifestations of somatoform disorders.

Options:
A. Briquet's disorder.
B. Depersonalisation.
C. Dysthymia.
D. Generalised anxiety disorder.
E. Hypochondriacal disorder.
F. Mixed dissociative disorder.
G. Neurasthenia.
H. Somatisation disorder.
I. Somatoform autonomic dysfunction.

Each option may be used once, more than once or not at all.

Lead-in: A 35-year-old male has a two-year history of physical symptoms for which no adequate physical explanation has been found. He keeps attending doctors in spite of investigations and reassurance and has some degree of impairment of social and family functioning.

For each of the following scenarios, choose the most likely ICD-10 disorder above that is occurring.

Stems: 120.1 The patient's main concern is multiple somatic symptoms and their individual effects. He asks for treatment to remove these symptoms.

120.2 The patient is concerned about an underlying progressive and serious disease process and asks for investigation to confirm the underlying disease. The patient fears medications and their side-effects.

120.3 He has a six-month history of persistent troublesome palpitations, sweating, tremor and flushing, and he has a chronic precordial pain. Even though he was investigated and repeatedly reassured that there was no evidence of ischaemic heart disease, he does not trust this and is preoccupied about the possibility of some serious disorder of his heart.

Question 121. Paraphilias

Theme: Paraphilias.

Options:

A.	Exhibitionism.	G.	Polymorphously perverse.
B.	Fetishism.	H.	Public masturbation.
C.	Frotteurism.	I.	Sadomasochism.
D.	Necrophilia.	J.	Transvestism.
E.	Paedophilia.	K.	Voyeurism.
F.	Partialism.	L.	Zoophilia.

Each option may be used once, more than once or not at all.

Lead-in: For each of the following individuals, choose the term above that best describes his paraphilia.

Stems:

121.1   A 34-year-old man gets pleasure from imagining the reaction of a woman who lives across the road were he to reveal to her that he masturbates while observing her showering most nights via his telescope.

121.2   A 60-year-old man achieves his sexual gratification by rubbing his genitals against the thighs of young women on crowded underground trains while travelling to work.

121.3   A 27-year-old man fantasises about women's feet and will only achieve orgasm during sexual intercourse with his girlfriend if he can see her feet during the act.

121.4   A 33-year-old man repeatedly hides behind bushes until he identifies an appropriate female approaching. When he sees one, he steps out in front of her with his trousers down and masturbates openly.

Question 122. *Physical signs*

Theme: Physical signs.

Options: A.   Barlow's sign.   E.   Omega sign.
               B.   Chvostek's sign.   F.   Russell's sign.
               C.   Hoffman's sign.   G.   Trendelenburg's sign.
               D.   Kernig's sign.   H.   Trousseau's sign.

Each option may be used once, more than once or not at all.

Lead-in: For each of the following patients, choose the required
               number of signs above that are most likely to be
               positive/present. Unless instructed otherwise, choose one
               sign per patient.

Stems: 122.1   A 19-year-old woman has excessive concern about
                       her weight. Although she is only slightly
                       overweight, it is revealed that she frequently eats
                       very large amounts of food in an uncontrollable
                       fashion and then induces vomiting to prevent
                       weight gain. Her blood chemistry reveals a slightly
                       lowered potassium.

               122.2   A 72-year-old man presents with depressed mood
                       present for the last four months. He has lost weight
                       and tends to stay in bed for most of the day. He
                       complains about his poor sleep and constipation. He
                       looks worried and eventually admits to having
                       marked guilt symptoms for some minor
                       transgressions in the past. His blood chemistry is
                       unremarkable.

               122.3   A 23-year-old man has an acute onset of second
                       person auditory hallucinations. He is disoriented
                       and drowsy. His family call the general practitioner
                       when he starts vomiting. When examined, the
                       patient is lying in a darkened room and complains
                       of headache. In hospital, his cerebrospinal fluid is
                       found to have increased cells and protein.

               122.4   A 60-year-old man has developed intellectual
                       impairment over the last three years. His mood
                       tends to be somewhat labile and his poor
                       concentration is evident during the interview. His
                       family have noticed a decline in interests over the
                       last few years. Blood chemistry reveals a low serum
                       calcium and raised phosphate. *(Choose two options)*

Question 123. Disorders in old age

Theme: Disorders in old age.

Options: A.   Alcohol dependence syndrome.
              B.   Charles Bonnet syndrome.
              C.   Delirium, unspecified.
              D.   Delusional disorder.
              E.   Depressive episode.
              F.   Dysthymia.
              G.   Late-onset schizophrenia.
              H.   Manic episode.
              I.   Mixed affective episode.
              J.   Unspecified dementia.

Each option may be used once, more than once or not at all.

Lead-in: For each of the following patients, choose the most
              appropriate diagnosis above.

Stems: 123.1   A 70-year-old woman who lives alone is referred
                       for assessment because she has been shouting at
                       neighbours. She believes that they have been in
                       her house, making entrance by passing through
                       her front wall. On occasional she has seen a
                       'vision' of Saint Therese. There is no evidence of
                       flattening of affect or thought disorder. Her
                       memory and orientation are normal.

              123.2   A 65-year-old man shrugs when asked about his
                       mood but spends some time talking about his
                       constipation and poor energy. He is worried that
                       this may be cancer. He is sleeping poorly and
                       finds it difficult to stay sitting during the
                       interview. His memory and orientation appear
                       normal but his concentration is diminished.

              123.3   A 68-year-old woman is displaying marked
                       uncharacteristic irritability. She sleeps less during
                       the night than usual but still remains
                       exceptionally active during the day. She speaks
                       rapidly and refuses to see her doctor as she has
                       'very important things to accomplish'. Her
                       memory and orientation are normal.

Question 124. Organic disorders

Theme: Organic disorders.

Options: A.   Addison's disease.
               B.   Cardiovascular examination.
               C.   Cushing's syndrome.
               D.   Diabetes mellitus.
               E.   Glabella tap.
               F.   Hypoparathyroidism.
               G.   Hyperthyroidism.
               H.   Hypopituitrism.
               I.   Hypothyroidism.
               J.   Sleeping pulse rate.
               K.   Thyrotoxicosis.

Each option may be used once, more than once or not at all.

Lead-in: Choose the term above that best fits each of the following
               statements on endocrine disturbances that are commonly
               associated with neuropsychiatric manifestations.

Stems: 124.1   A young female is admitted for the treatment of
                        agitated depression. She also has hot sweaty
                        palms, tremor and tachycardia. This bedside
                        examination is a useful sign in distinguishing
                        between functional and organic disorder.

               124.2   In this endocrine disturbance, the psychiatric
                        features are related to the serum calcium level.

               124.3   Insidious onset of weakness, fatigue, weight loss,
                        gastrointestinal symptoms, depression, mild
                        cognitive impairment and hyperpigmentation on
                        the exposed areas and skin creases suggest this
                        endocrine disease.

Question 125. *Patterns of behaviour in personality disorders*

Theme: Patterns of behaviour in personality disorders.

Options: A.   Antisocial personality disorder.
                B.   Avoidant personality disorder.
                C.   Borderline personality disorder.
                D.   Histrionic personality disorder.
                E.   Narcissistic personality disorder.
                F.   Obsessive-compulsive personality disorder.
                G.   Paranoid personality disorder.
                H.   Schizoid personality disorder.
                I.   Schizotypal personality disorder.

Each option may be used once, more than once or not at all.

Lead-in: For each of the following sets of characteristics choose the most likely DSM-IV personality disorder above being described.

Stems: 125.1   This cluster C personality disorder is characterised by pervasive and excessive hypersensitivity to negative evaluation, social inhibition, feelings of inadequacy and social and occupational difficulties.

              125.2   The hallmarks of this cluster B personality disorder are pervasive and excessive instability of affect, unstable self-image and interpersonal relationships, impulsivity, and chronic feelings of emptiness

              125.3   This cluster A personality disorder is characterised by distrust and excessive suspiciousness expressed as a pervasive tendency to interpret the actions of others as deliberately deceiving, exploiting, threatening and demeaning to the individual.

Question 126. *Sleep disturbances in psychiatric disorders*

Theme: Sleep disturbances in psychiatric disorders.

Options: A.   Amphetamine.
               B.   Depressive disorder.
               C.   Eating disorders.
               D.   Ethanol.
               E.   Generalised anxiety disorder.
               F.   Heroin.
               G.   Morphine.
               H.   Nicotine.
               I.   Schizophrenia.

Each option may be used once, more than once or not at all.

Lead-in: For each of the following statements about sleep changes
               in psychiatric disorders, choose the phrase above that best
               fits the statement.

Stems: 126.1   In this psychiatric disorder changes in rapid eye
                        movement (REM) sleep or slow wave sleep are not
                        typically observed.

               126.2   In this psychiatric disorder there is strong
                        evidence of decreased slow wave sleep, decreased
                        delta (δ) wave activity, and an increased REM
                        percentage of total sleep.

               126.3   Withdrawal from this chemical agent may cause
                        increased REM density and/or increased amount
                        of REM sleep.

               126.4   Withdrawal from this chemical agent is
                        characterised by increases in total sleep and REM
                        sleep.

Question 127. Delirium

Theme: Delirium.

Options: A.   Cerebrovascular disease.
               B.   Cholinergic hypoactivity.
               C.   Cholinergic hyperactivity.
               D.   Dopamine hyperactivity.
               E.   Excessive alcohol use.
               F.   Immediate and short-term memory.
               G.   Immediate, short-term and long-term memory.
               H.   Intoxication due to prescribed medication.
               I.   Nocturnal arousal and daytime drowsiness.
               J.   Nocturnal drowsiness and daytime arousal.

Each option may be used once, more than once or not at all.

Lead-in: Choose the phrase above that best fits each of the
               following statements about delirium.

Stems: 127.1   This disturbance of sleep–wake cycle is very
                       common in delirium.

               127.2   This is the most common single cause of delirium
                       in the elderly.

               127.3   Alcohol withdrawal delirium is commonly
                       associated with this neurotransmitter abnormality.

               127.4   In delirium of moderate severity, these are the
                       most common memory functions affected.

Question 128. Hierarchical structure of diagnosis in ICD-10

Theme: Hierarchical structure of diagnosis in ICD-10.

Options: A.   Affective disorder.
          B.   Neurotic disorders.
          C.   Organic psychosis.
          D.   Schizophrenia and affective disorders are both at the same level.
          E.   Schizophrenia is above the affective disorders in the hierarchy.
          F.   The given diagnosis excludes the presence of symptoms of all higher members of the hierarchy.
          G.   The given diagnosis excludes the presence of symptoms of all lower members of the hierarchy.
          H.   The hierarchies are different to that of ICD-10.
          I.   The hierarchies are the same as that of ICD-10.

Each option may be used once only.

Lead-in: ICD-10 follows a hierarchical structure of diagnosis. Choose the phrase above that best fits the following statements about this hierarchical structure.

Stems: 128.1   In general the hierarchical structure of diagnosis has this characteristic regarding the exclusion of symptoms at different levels of the hierarchy.

          128.2   Schizophrenia and affective disorder in the hierarchy of ICD-10 have this relationship.

          128.3   These disorders come at the bottom of the ICD-10 hierarchy.

          128.4   This is true of the hierarchies of other international classification systems compared to the hierarchy of ICD-10.

Question 129. DSM-IV personality disorder criteria

Theme: DSM-IV personality disorder criteria.

Options: A.   Affective instability.   F.   Miserliness.
              B.   Constricted affect.   G.   Sensitive to criticism.
              C.   Impulsivity.   H.   Stubbornness.
              D.   Irresponsibility.   I.   Suggestibility.
              E.   Lacks empathy.   J.   Suspiciousness.

Each option may be used once, more than once or not at all.

Lead-in: For each of the following personality disorders, **select
              two traits** above that are listed in its DSM-IV
              diagnostic criteria.

Stems: 129.1   Antisocial personality disorder.

              129.2   Obsessive-compulsive personality disorder.

              129.3   Paranoid personality disorder.

              129.4   Borderline personality disorder.

Question 130. Sleep disorders and parasomnias

Theme: Sleep disorders and parasomnias.

Options: A.   Advanced sleep-phase syndrome.
                B.   Bruxism.
                C.   Delayed sleep-phase syndrome.
                D.   Entrainment failure.
                E.   Idiopathic hypersomnia.
                F.   Kline-Levin syndrome.
                G.   Narcolepsy.
                H.   Nightmare.
                I.   Night terror.
                J.   Pickwickian syndrome.
                K.   Sleep myoclonus.
                L.   Somnambulism.

Each option may be used once, more than once or not at all.

Lead-in: For each of the following vignettes, select the likeliest sleep
                disorder or parasomnia above that is occurring.

Stems: 130.1   A man complains of feeling very tired during the
                         day and finds himself irresistibly falling asleep for
                         periods at work. He often hears his voice spoken
                         aloud when going to sleep and has noted falling to
                         the ground when he laughs at a particularly
                         funny joke.

                130.2   A young man has periods lasting about two days
                         when he sleeps for long periods both night and
                         day. When awake, he tends to be irritable and
                         reports occasionally hearing his name spoken
                         aloud by a female voice.

                130.3   A young female has marked somnolence during
                         the day. She is noted to be markedly overweight
                         and has cyanotic periods.

                130.4   Soon after a girl child is put to bed, she
                         occasionally screams aloud, upsetting her parents.
                         Occasionally she wets the bed at the same time,
                         but when questioned about the event, she
                         invariably says that she does not remember what
                         has happened.

Question 131. Alcohol use disorders

Theme: Alcohol use disorders.

Options: A.   Family history of bipolar disorder.
               B.   Family history of female alcoholics.
               C.   Family history of male alcoholics.
               D.   Higher ratio of water to fat than in the male body.
               E.   Lower activity of alcohol dehydrogenase in the gastric mucosa.
               F.   Lower activity of alcohol dehydrogenase in the liver.
               G.   M:F = 2:1.
               H.   M:F = 4:1.
               I.   M:F = 5:1.
               J.   Previous sexual abuse is more common than in the general population.
               K.   Previous sexual abuse is not raised when compared to the general population.

Each option may be used once, more than once or not at all.

Lead-in: A 50-year-old woman has a two-year history of heavy alcohol consumption and has physical signs of dependence. Answer the following questions about her condition with the most appropriate statement above.

Stems: 131.1   When compared to a man, she is likely to have a higher peak blood level for a given dose of ethanol. This is most likely to be due to which mechanism?

               131.2   What is the ratio of male to female alcoholics seen in psychiatric practice?

               131.3   What finding in her family history is most likely to be present?

               131.4   What is the relationship of childhood sexual abuse to alcohol dependence?

Question 132. Culture-bound syndromes

Theme: Culture-bound syndromes.

Options:

A.	*Amok.*	G.	*Locura.*
B.	*Bouffée délirante.*	H.	*Mal de ojo.*
C.	*Cathard.*	I.	*Piblokto.*
D.	*Dhat.*	J.	*Susto.*
E.	*Koro.*	K.	*Windigo.*
F.	*Latah.*	L.	*Zar.*

Each option may be used once, more than once or not at all.

Lead-in: For each of the following patient vignettes, choose the most likely culture-bound syndrome above it illustrates.

Stems:

132.1 A Polynesian male is observed to show a sudden onset of uncharacteristic psychomotor excitement with marked violence and paranoid symptoms.

132.2 A Malaysian women presents with a sudden onset of marked anxiety that her nipples will retract into her body and cause her death.

132.3 A native North American male is apprehended after an onset of uncharacteristic behaviour in which he tried to eat his neighbour.

132.4 A Mexican woman presents with anxiety symptoms following being mugged a year previously. She states that her symptoms are a result of her soul having left her body following the trauma.

Question 133. Depression in the postpartum period

Theme: Depression in the postpartum period.

Options: A.   Depression in both the postpartum and non-
                    postpartum periods.
               B.   Depression in the postpartum period only.
               C.   Depressive episode.
               D.   Longer duration.
               E.   Maternity blues.
               F.   Non-Western societies.
               G.   Post-natal depression.
               H.   Shorter duration.
               I.   Western societies.

Each option may be used once, more than once or not at all.

Lead-in: A 20-year-old woman delivered her first baby six weeks
               ago. This was an unplanned pregnancy. Her partner
               deserted her when he learned that she was pregnant. Her
               parents are staunch Catholics. For the last two weeks, she
               is more weepy and irritable. She is extremely concerned
               about the well-being of her child and thinks that she is not
               a good mother. She also has sleep disturbances, vegetative
               symptoms of depression and fleeting thoughts of self-
               harm. There is no positive family history of affective
               disorder and she has no previous history of affective
               disorder.

               *Answer the following questions about this woman with depressive
               symptoms in the postpartum period with the most appropriate
               phrase from the above.*

Stems: 133.1   What is her most likely ICD-10 diagnosis?

               133.2   For what duration is she likely to have this
                       condition?

               133.3   She is at increased risk of further depressive
                       episodes during which period(s)?

               133.4   Ethnographic studies indicate that depression
                       occurring in the postpartum period only is rare in
                       which societies?

Question 134. Psychotherapy

Theme: Psychotherapy.

Options: A.   Behavioural therapy.
                B.   Brief psychodynamic psychotherapy.
                C.   Cognitive-analytic therapy.
                D.   Cognitive therapy.
                E.   Counselling.
                F.   Gestalt therapy.
                G.   Interpersonal psychotherapy.
                H.   Primal therapy.
                I.   Psychoanalytic psychotherapy.
                J.   Transactional psychotherapy.

Each option may be used once, more than once or not at all.

Lead-in: For each of the following descriptions of psychotherapy,
                select the therapy above that is being used.

Stems: 134.1   A 33-year-old woman develops depression after
                         losing her job. Having diagnosed the individual, the
                         therapist assigns her the sick role and informs her
                         that they will have sixteen sessions in total.
                         Between them, they agree that her symptoms have
                         arisen from a role transition. Therapy involves
                         helping her to address her current relationships
                         with others to assist her in this transition.

                134.2   A 28-year-old man with dysthymic disorder begins
                         psychotherapy. A total of sixteen sessions is agreed.
                         The therapist conducts exploration of interactions
                         within present relationships, and considers
                         transference issues. The therapist encourages free
                         association from the patient at times and pays
                         attention to his defence mechanisms.

                134.3   A 48-year-old woman has generalised anxiety
                         symptoms. She and the therapist agree to meet for
                         eight sessions. The therapist makes efforts to build
                         a therapeutic relationship with her. She is allowed
                         to express emotions freely in the session. Much
                         focus is placed on her current difficulties in her
                         social situation. An attempt is made to discover her
                         strengths and how she can use these to overcome
                         some of these difficulties.

Question 135. Psychoanalysis

Theme: Psychoanalysis.

Options: A.   Abreaction.
             B.   Acting out.
             C.   Countertransference.
             D.   Dissociative anaesthesia and sensory loss.
             E.   Dissociative motor disorder.
             F.   Free association.
             G.   Inductive questioning.
             H.   Role-play.
             I.   Somatisation disorder.
             J.   Transference.

Each option may be used once, more than once or not at all.

Lead-in: A 20-year-old woman had suddenly developed aphonia, for which no organic reason could be identified. A psychoanalytic psychotherapist treated her. During the therapy, she became angry with the therapist as he reminded her of her father.

Choose the phrase above about her condition and treatment that best answers each of the following questions.

Stems: 135.1   What is the most likely ICD-10 diagnosis of her illness?

             135.2   Which therapeutic method is her therapist most likely to employ?

             135.3   The emotional reliving of her past trauma is termed what?

             135.4   Of what is the patient's unwarranted behaviour towards the therapist during the treatment an example?

Question 136. *Mood disorders in DSM-IV*

Theme: Mood disorders in DSM-IV.

Options: A.   Bipolar I Disorder.
                B.   Bipolar II Disorder.
                C.   Bipolar Disorder NOS*.
                D.   Cyclothymic Disorder.
                E.   Depressive Disorder NOS*.
                F.   Dysthymic Disorder.
                G.   Hypomanic Episode.
                H.   Major Depressive Episode.
                I.   Major Depressive Disorder.
                J.   Manic Episode.
                K.   Mixed Episode.
                L.   Substance-induced Mood Disorder.

Each option may be used once, more than once or not at all.

Lead-in: For each of the following patients, select the DSM-IV
                diagnosis above that best denotes his/her condition.

Stems: 136.1   A 27-year-old man has a history over the last two
                       years of numerous periods when he experiences
                       symptoms fulfilling criteria for a hypomanic
                       episode. During this time he has also experienced
                       numerous spells of depressive symptoms, but
                       these have never met criteria for a full depressive
                       episode. The longest time he has been without
                       symptoms has been one month.

              136.2   A 36-year old man has a ten-day history of
                       symptoms fulfilling criteria for a manic episode,
                       but is noted to have marked depressive symptoms
                       which do not fulfil criteria for a major depressive
                       episode.

              136.3   A 28-year-old woman develops symptoms
                       fulfilling criteria for a hypomanic episode while
                       on antidepressant therapy. These symptoms
                       resolve after the antidepressant is stopped. This
                       treatment was for a single episode of major
                       depression six months ago that resolved
                       completely.

*Not otherwise specified

Question 137. ICD-10 classification of anxiety disorders

Theme: ICD-10 classification of anxiety disorders.

Options: A.   Agoraphobia.
B.   Animal phobia.
C.   Fifth character.
D.   Fourth character.
E.   Other phobic anxiety disorders.
F.   Phobia anxiety disorder.
G.   Social phobia.
H.   Specific phobia.
I.   Third character.

Each option may be used once, more than once or not at all.

Lead-in: Choose the phrase above that best answers each of the following questions about the ICD-10 classification of anxiety disorders.

Stems: 137.1   *Anthropophobia* is included under which phobia?

137.2   If the distinction between social phobia and agoraphobia is very difficult, precedence should be given to which phobia?

137.3   In agoraphobia, the presence or absence of panic disorder is recorded by means of which character in ICD-10?

137.4   Claustrophobia is included under which phobia?

Question 138. Diagnosing personality disorders using DSM-IV

Theme: Diagnosing personality disorders using DSM-IV.

Options: A. Antisocial.   G. Narcissistic.
              B. Avoidant.   H. Obsessive-compulsive.
              C. Borderline.   I. Paranoid.
              D. Dependent.   J. Passive-aggressive.
              E. Depressive.   K. Schizoid.
              F. Histrionic.   L. Schizotypal.

Each option may be used once, more than once or not at all.

Lead-in: A 28-year-old man comes reluctantly to your psychiatric
               outpatient clinic accompanied by his mother. He explains
               that his boss at work has ordered him to get himself 'sorted
               out'. *Choose the required number of personality disorders above to
               answer the following.*

Stems: 138.1   He hands you a perfunctory letter from his
                       general practitioner that has been opened. It
                       reads: '? Axis II condition. ? Cluster B' *What
                       conditions does his general practitioner suspect? (Four
                       answers)*

               138.2   You note that the patient appears quite suspicious
                       of you. He has a constricted affect and states that
                       he fears you will use any information he gives you
                       against him. His mother notes that these traits
                       have been present since he was about 16, and
                       that he tends to have few contacts outside his
                       immediate family. *What are the main personality
                       disorders you would consider in your differential
                       diagnosis at this stage? (Three answers)*

               138.3   As the interview progresses his mother convinces
                       him to speak to you, although he remains clearly
                       anxious and suspicious. The patient admits he has
                       had difficulties at work, being unable to handle
                       the frequent jokes co-workers make about his
                       unusual dress sense. His manner of speech is
                       vague but he gets across his belief to you that he
                       may have a sixth sense about things that will
                       happen in the future. His mother notes that he
                       had similar difficulties in secondary school. *What
                       is your working diagnosis now? (One answer)*

Question 139. Complications of excessive alcohol

Theme: Complications of excessive alcohol.

Options: A.   Acute vitamin B deficiencies.
                B.   Hyperglycaemia.
                C.   Hypotension.
                D.   Invariably with abnormal liver functions tests.
                E.   Normal liver functions tests.
                F.   Polyneuropathy.
                G.   Reactive hypoglycaemia.
                H.   Subdural haematoma.
                I.   Supraventicular arrhythmias.
                J.   Ventricular conduction defects.

Each option may be used once, more than once or not at all.

Lead-in: A 50-year-old man has been drinking 40 units of alcohol
                every week for the last four years. For each of the
                following questions about possible complications from his
                drinking, choose the most appropriate answer above.

Stems: 139.1   Disturbance of consciousness with unilateral facial
                       weakness in him must raise the suspicion of which
                       condition?

              139.2   The occurrence of steatosis is possibly associated
                       with which profile of liver function tests?

              139.3   Individuals with chronic alcoholism are prone to
                       develop which condition following a
                       carbohydrate-rich meal?

              139.4   Bouts of excessive drinking cause which effect on
                       the cardiovascular system?

Question 140. Dementia syndromes

Theme: Dementia syndromes.

Options: A.   Alzheimer's disease.
            B.   Binswanger's disease.
            C.   Creutzfeldt-Jakob disease.
            D.   Dementia with Lewy bodies.
            E.   Frontotemporal dementia.
            F.   Huntington's disease.
            G.   Multi-infarct dementia.
            H.   Normal pressure hydrocephalus.
            I.   Parkinson's disease.
            J.   Pick's disease.

Each option may be used once, more than once or not at all.

Lead-in: For each of the following patients, choose the type of dementia above from which he/she is most likely to be suffering.

Stems: 140.1   A 59-year-old man has progressive memory impairment. His insight is good and he feels his major difficulties are the associated ataxia and dysarthria, all of which worsened in distinct phases. He has difficulty swallowing and has a brisk jaw jerk. He has a history of hypertension. MRI shows bilateral subcortical white matter low attenuation while the cortex appears normal.

140.2   A 56-year-old woman has mild memory impairment. She has poor insight and has become disinhibited in her behaviour, appearing to be in constant good form. MRI shows enlarged ventricles frontally and marked atrophy of the frontal and temporal lobes. After her death, histology shows argyrophilic inclusion bodies in her neurons.

140.3   A 48-year-old woman has mild memory impairment. She is noticed to be apathetic and to be much less spontaneous. She walks in a shuffling, stiff-legged fashion. She has recently developed intermittent urinary incontinence. She has a history of meningitis. MRI shows enlarged ventricles.

Question 141. *Bipolar affective disorder*

Theme: Bipolar affective disorder.

Options: A.   Acceleration and retardation.
              B.   Bipolar affective disorder I.
              C.   Bipolar affective disorder II.
              D.   Circumstantiality.
              E.   Hepatitis.
              F.   Hypothyroidism.
              G.   Pruritic rash.
              H.   Successful prophylaxis.
              I.   Tangentiality.
              J.   Unstable course of bipolar disorder.

Each option may be used once, more than once or not at all.

Lead-in: A 40-year-old man has a history of bipolar affective
              disorder. He has had three episodes of mania, one with
              psychotic symptoms, and two episodes of depression of
              mild severity. He is on valproate monotherapy. He now
              exhibits mild depression.

              *For each of the following questions about his condition and its
              pharmacotherapy, select the phrase above that best answers it.*

Stems: 141.1   What is the characteristic disturbance(s) in his
                     flow of thinking over the course of his illness to
                     date?

              141.2   Which possible serious adverse effect may develop
                     after adding lamotrigine to his current treatment?

              141.3   What is the possible outcome of adding a selective
                     serotonin reuptake inhibitor to his treatment?

              141.4   How would this patient's bipolar affective

Question 142. *Psychopathology of endocrine disorders*

Theme: Psychopathology of endocrine disorders.

Options:

A.	Acromegaly.	F.	Hypoparathyroidism.
B.	Adrenocortical deficiency.	G.	Hypothyroidism.
C.	Cushing's syndrome.	H.	Insulinoma.
D.	Hyperparathyroidism.	I.	Phaeochromocytoma.
E.	Hyperthyroidism.	J.	Steroid treatment.

Each option may be used once, more than once or not at all.

Lead-in: For each of the following patients with endocrine disorders, choose the condition above that is the most likely cause of his/her symptoms.

Stems: 142.1 A 63-year-old man presents with elated mood that is frequently labile. He is occasionally irritable and his family have noticed him to be markedly apathetic over the last year. He complains of pins and needles in his hands, and headache. On examination he has greasy skin with an enlarged jaw and feet. On investigation, the patient has impaired glucose tolerance and is hypertensive.

142.2 A 37-year-old woman presents with marked depression with melancholic features. She has had suicidal ideation and has heard a male voice telling her that she is 'evil'. She complains of poor energy. She is noted to have a proximal myopathy, bruising and central obesity. On investigation, she is hyperglycaemic and hypertensive.

142.3 A 56-year-old man is noticed to be markedly agitated and anxious. He denies sustained depressed mood but complains of waking earlier than usual. His family have noticed increased irritability and state that his appetite is much better than it had been in the past. He appears to have lost weight and is sweating on examination. Blood glucose levels are within normal levels and his blood pressure is normal, although a sinus tachycardia is present.

Question 143. *Correlates of outcome in schizophrenia*

Theme: Correlates of outcome in schizophrenia.

Options: A.   Affective symptoms.   F.   Paranoid symptoms.
                B.   Hyperprolactinaemia.   G.   Parkinsonism.
                C.   Male sex.   H.   Poor insight.
                D.   Married.   I.   Unemployment.
                E.   Older age of onset.   J.   Ventricular
                                                    enlargement.

Each option may be used once, more than once or not at all.

Lead-in: For each of the following questions put to you, choose the
                required number of factors above that are most associated
                with the outcome in question.

Stems: 143.1   A 23-year-old man has been newly diagnosed as
                       having schizophrenia. At a meeting with the
                       family, his mother asks what factors are associated
                       with good outcome in schizophrenia. *(Choose four
                       options.)*

               143.2   His father then asks what factors are associated
                       with poor outcome in schizophrenia.
                       (Choose four options.)

               143.3   Later, the community psychiatric nurse wonders if
                       he will take any medication prescribed after
                       leaving hospital. She asks you what possible factors
                       might be associated with non-concordance. *(Choose
                       three options.)*

               143.4   The ward manager is worried about the patient's
                       safety and asks you what factors are associated
                       with risk of suicide in schizophrenia.
                       (Choose four options.)

Question 144. Sequelae of alcohol abuse

Theme: Sequelae of alcohol abuse.

Options: A.   Alcohol-induced amnesia.
                  B.   Alcohol-induced psychosis.
                  C.   Alcoholic hallucinosis.
                  D.   Central pontine myelinolysis.
                  E.   Korsakoff syndrome.
                  F.   Hepatocerebral degeneration.
                  G.   Marchiafava-Bignami syndrome.
                  H.   Wernicke's encephalopathy.

Each option may be used once only.

Lead-in: Each of the following patients has a long-standing history of alcohol abuse. From their symptoms, choose the syndrome above that is most likely to be occurring.

Stems: 144.1   A 57-year-old man is unable to walk and spasticity is noted in his limbs. Mental state examination is difficult as his speech is very indistinct but suggests the presence of a dementia. MRI (magnetic resonance imaging) shows demyelination of the corpus callosum.

                 144.2   A 73-year-old woman has an ataxic gait. Nystagmus is noted on examination. She is noted to be disoriented in place and time on mental state examination. CT (computerised tomography) reveals brain tissue atrophy consistent with her age.

                 144.3   A 38-year-old woman is tremulous and agitated. She is sweating and has raised blood pressure. She is disoriented in time and place and reports seeing leprechauns brandishing knives under the table. CT is unremarkable.

                 144.4   A 62-year-old man with alcoholic cirrhosis is being treated in hospital. When his hyponatraemia is corrected, the patient develops quadriplegia and difficulties with moving his tongue. His jaw jerk is normal and his voice is hoarse. MRI reveals some focal demyelination.

Question 145. Movement disorders

Theme: Movement disorders.

Options: A.   Caudate nucleus.
               B.   Frontal lobe.
               C.   Globus pallidus.
               D.   Nigro-striatum.
               E.   No consistant pathology.
               F.   Pre-frontal cortex.
               G.   Putamen.
               H.   Striatum.
               I.   Subthalamic nucleus.
               J.   Thalamus.

Each option may be used once, more than once or not at all.

Lead-in: Lesions of which of the above cause the following clinical
               syndromes?

Stems: 145.1   An adult male exhibits slow, irregular, writhing
                       involuntary movements occurring about the long
                       axis of his left upper and lower limbs, associated
                       with hypertonia.

               145.2   An adult female exhibits recurrent rapid,
                       flapping, violent involuntary movements,
                       commonly associated with normal tone.

               145.3   An adult male exhibits rapid, repetitive,
                       stereotyped involuntary movements of synergistic
                       muscle groups, associated with normal tone.

               145.4   An adult male exhibits irregular, rapid, jerking,
                       quasi-purposive involuntary movements,
                       associated with normal tone.

Question 146. *Psychotic and related disorders in ICD-10*

Theme: Psychotic and related disorders in ICD-10.

Options: A.   Acute polymorphic psychotic disorder.
B.   Acute schizophrenia-like disorder.
C.   Delusional disorder.
D.   Induced delusional disorder.
E.   Paranoid schizophrenia.
F.   Schizoaffective disorder, depressive type.
G.   Schizoaffective disorder, manic type.
H.   Schizoid personality disorder.
I.   Schizotypal disorder.
J.   Simple schizophrenia.

Each option may be used once, more than once or not at all.

Lead-in: For each of the following vignettes, select the most appropriate diagnosis above.

Stems: 146.1   A 34-year-old woman is admitted with persistent third-person commentary auditory hallucinations. Her speech at times is irrelevant in content. The patient also believes she can speak to aliens from 'Riga 7'. Collateral history reveals she has had these hallucinations for the last two months. A few days after these began the patient was noted to be overactive, over-talkative and sleeping less, but was markedly irritable. These mood symptoms continue to be evident.

146.2   A 78-year-old man is seen on a domiciliary visit. For the last eighteen months, he believes certain programmes on the television are referring to him in particular. He has low mood but this is recent according to the patient. The patient is very alert and oriented and objectively appears slightly sad. His speech is coherent and relevant.

146.3   A 28-year-old woman is admitted following the acute onset of ideas that members of the Real IRA might be stalking her. These symptoms settle rapidly in hospital. The patient's speech tends to be circumstantial. She remains aloof from other patients and staff while in hospital and insists on wearing two skirts and a pair of trousers, which she says is her normal style. Collateral from neighbours suggests that she has always been considered peculiar but generally copes well.

Question 147. Neuropsychiatric sequelae of multiple sclerosis

Theme: Neuropsychiatric sequelae of multiple sclerosis.

Options:
A. Chromosome 2.
B. Chromosome 6.
C. Chromosome 9.
D. Cognitive impairment.
E. Generalised anxiety disorder.
F. Major depressive episode.
G. Manic episode.
H. Rapidly progressive dementia.
I. Sensorimotor impairment.
J. Slowly progressive dementia.

Each option may be used once, more than once or not at all.

Lead-in: A 30-year-old female has optic neuritis, diplopia, ataxia, sensory and motor disturbances in her limbs. These symptoms have had a relapsing and remitting course for the last few years.

Answer each of the following questions about her condition using the most appropriate of the above phrases.

Stems:
147.1 Which is the most common psychiatric disorder she is likely to develop?

147.2 If she develops euphoria, with what finding does this generally correlate?

147.3 An association between her condition and the HLA region of which chromosome has been described?

147.4 If she develops dementia, how will this typically progress?

Question 148. Sequelae of vitamin deficiencies

Theme: Sequelae of vitamin deficiencies.

Options: A. Vitamin A.   G. Vitamin D.
                B. Vitamin B_1 (thiamine).   H. Vitamin E.
                C. Vitamin B_2 (riboflavin).   I. Vitamin K.
                D. Vitamin B_6 (pyridoxine).   J. Folic acid (folate).
                E. Vitamin B_{12}.   K. Nicotinic acid (niacin).
                F. Vitamin C.   L. Pantothenic acid.

Each option may be used once, more than once or not at all.

Lead-in: For each of the following patients, select which vitamin
               deficiency is most likely to have caused his/her symptoms.

Stems: 148.1   A 68-year-old man weighing 55 kg is admitted to
                       the general hospital. He is noted to have marked
                       lability of mood, sometimes stating tearfully that he
                       sees 'no reason to go on'. He complains of ongoing
                       diarrhoea and intermittent headaches. Physical
                       examination reveals skin lesions and glossitis. Blood
                       results are unremarkable. Collateral history suggests
                       very poor living conditions.

               148.2   A 31-year-old woman weighing 60 kg is admitted to
                       the general hospital. She is markedly disoriented in
                       time and place. Physical examination demonstrates
                       a staggering gait and evidence of a sixth nerve palsy
                       on visual tracking. Blood results confirm she is
                       pregnant. Collateral history reveals that she has
                       been vomiting severely over the last few weeks.

               148.3   A 72-year-old woman weighing 57 kg is admitted to
                       the psychiatric unit. She appears depressed and
                       describes auditory hallucinations. She complains of
                       poor appetite and lethargy. Physical examination
                       reveals altered proprioception. Blood results show a
                       macrocytic anaemia and decreased alkaline
                       phosphatase levels. Collateral history is unavailable.

               148.4   A 36-year-old man weighing 82 kg is seen in
                       psychiatric outpatients. He is noted to have
                       depressed mood of moderate severity. He states
                       that he has a history of epilepsy that is well
                       controlled with phenytoin. Physical examination is
                       unremarkable. Blood results later reveal a
                       macrocytic anaemia. Collateral history is
                       unavailable.

Question 149. *The electroencephalogram (EEG)*

Theme: The electroencephalogram (EEG).

Options: A.   Decreased α activity.
               B.   Decreased β activity.
               C.   Decreased δ activity.
               D.   Decreased θ activity.
               E.   Decreased λ activity.
               F.   Increased α activity.
               G.   Increased β activity.
               H.   Increased δ activity.
               I.   Increased θ activity.
               J.   Increased λ activity.
               K.   Three-hertz spikes and waves.
               L.   Triphasic sharp wave complexes.

Each option may be used once, more than once or not at all.

Lead-in: For each of the following individuals, select all appropriate
               EEG findings above that one would **normally** expect to
               find.

Stems: 149.1   A 36-year-old male with Creutzfeld-Jakob disease.

               149.2   A 47-year-old female with Huntington's disease.

               149.3   A 23-year-old male on chlordiazepoxide therapy.

               149.4   A 27-year-old female receiving lithium therapy
                       with levels in the therapeutic range.

Question 150. Phenotypic similarities between Axis I and Axis II disorders

Theme: Phenotypic similarities between Axis I and Axis II disorders.

Options:
A. Avoidant behaviour and shyness.
B. Dependency.
C. Elation.
D. Hypochondriasis and inflexibility.
E. Impulsiveness and mood swings.
F. Negative symptoms.
G. Positive symptoms.
H. Proneness to depressed mood and self-destruction.
I. Suspiciousness.

Each option may be used once, more than once or not at all.

Lead-in: Some DSM-IV Axis II disorders are considered as minor variants of an Axis I disorder as they share common symptoms. For each of the following parings of minor and major variants, select the symptom(s) above that they share.

Stems: 150.1 Narcissistic personality disorder is a minor variant of bipolar affective disorder.

150.2 Avoidant personality disorder is a minor variant of social phobia.

150.3 Antisocial personality disorder is a minor variant of bipolar affective disorder.

150.4 Dependent personality disorder is a minor variant of panic disorder with agoraphobia.

Answers

Psychology and Human Development EMIs

1. Operant conditioning
1.1 **B.** Hence there is a consistent responding. **[D. p419t]**
1.2 **D.** The response is steady in order to get a reward when it is available. **[D. p419t]**
1.3 **H.** As reinforcement has occurred at random intervals. **[D. p419t]**

2. Jean Piaget
2.1 **D.** During the sensorimotor stage, a number of significant concepts are developed including the child's concept of space and causality. **[D. p402–5]**
2.2 **A.** The other four characteristic behaviour patterns are imitations, graphic imagery, mental image and verbal evocation of events not occurring at the time. **[D. p402–5]**
2.3 **A.** As in 2.2 above. **[D. p402–5]**
2.4 **D.** This is object permanence. **[D. p402–5]**

3. Concepts of motivation
3.1 **H.** As the Yerkes-Dodson curve suggests, individuals tend to perform best with some, but not excessive, anxiety. Note: the authors do not recommend this SHO's study plan. **[B. p9]**
3.2 **E.** Maslow's hierarchy of needs indicates that there are some basic needs that must be satisfied before more lofty desires can be entertained. Self-actualisation is at the pinnacle of this pyramid, while food, shelter and other basic needs are at the base. **[J. p118–19]**
3.3 **G.** This is another intrinsic motivation theory: the action brings its own integral reward. **[B. p8–9]**
3.4 **B.** There is inconsistency between two of his beliefs: that he is a good psychiatrist, and that psychiatrists should have the MRCPsych. He is thus motivated to change one of these beliefs to resolve this inconsistency. **[J. p361–2]**

4. Aggression
4.1 **B.** This is based on Freudian psychological theory. However, available evidence fails to support the catharsis hypothesis. **[T. p97–111]**
4.2 **J.** This technique works well when non-aggressive behaviour is rewarded. **[T. p97–111]**
4.3 **C.** Fostering empathy has also been found to be beneficial with pre-school boys to reduce unruly behaviour. **[T. p97–111]**

4.4   **A.** This is a self-survival act to reduce injury to the organism. **[T. p97–111]**

5. Perception
5.1   **H.** Several studies have proved this consistently. **[Y. p208–16]**
5.2   **B.** It is likely that at least a basic level of depth perception is innate. **[Y. p208–16]**
5.3   **G.** If the size constancy is maintained, then the person in the Ames room will not change in size. **[Y. p208–16]**
5.4   **D.** In adaptation, the actual number of sensory messages sent to the brain is decreased, but when the message reaches the brain the orientation response occurs normally. **[Y. p208–16]**

6. Operant conditioning principles
6.1   **F.** This is not continuous reinforcement, since he gets his wages intermittently. It is fixed interval since the reward comes regularly every two weeks. (Note: all characters described in this book are fictional; any similarity to real individuals is purely coincidental) **[L. p121]**
6.2   **C.** While this is a form of self-administered aversive conditioning, the term that describes it most closely is *covert sensitisation* since the aversive event takes place in the individual's imagination. **[K. p3]**
6.3   **A.** Leaving aside the ethical concerns about this situation, it clearly is an attempt at aversion conditioning with a real aversive event. **[L. p126]**
6.4   **J.** This is again partial reinforcement, this time with a variable ratio schedule as is gambling: the more often you partake, the more often you 'win', but the gaps between these events varies greatly. It is highly resistant to extinction. **[L. p120–1]**

7. Lobar functions
7.1   **D.** Motor cortex involvement can result in hemiparesis and dysphasia. **[B. p283–5]**
7.2   **A.** Prosopagnosia and right/left disorientation suggests left parietal lobe involvement. Bilateral astereognosis suggests bilateral involvement. **[T. p283–5]**

8. Developmental and hereditary disorders
8.1   **D.** This syndrome is due to X chromosome heteromorphism. **[D. p872–6]**
8.2   **E.** The gene is located on chromosome 4 and the disorder is transmitted in an autosomal dominant fashion. **[D. p872–6]**
8.3   **A.** It is an autosomal dominant disease with partial penetrance. **[D. p872–6]**
8.4   **D.** The better-known manifestation of fragile X syndrome. **[D. p872–6]**

9. Concepts of aggression

9.1 **J.** This is one of Freud's modifications of his theories. Aggression need not be expressed physically: impulses can be sublimated by channelling such energies into socially acceptable pursuits. [**L. p99–100**]

9.2 **B.** This is a contribution of ethology: Lorenz suggested actions such as begging or smiling are examples of such appeasement rituals. [**L. p100–1**]

9.3 **E.** This theory has been criticised because of the pertinent observation that frustration does not always lead to aggression. [**L. p101–2**]

9.4 **C.** The idea is that the individual's identity is lost in the group and there are pressures to conform to the group's actions. [**J. p429–30**]

10. Concepts of classical and operant conditioning

10.1 **I.** Since the behaviours being rewarded are only those that resemble more and more closely the required outcome. [**B. p3**]

10.2 **D.** He may push it again intermittently after rest (partial recovery). [**M. p33**]

10.3 **L.** The light is acting as the conditioned stimulus and is removed before the unconditioned stimulus of the shock is presented. The conditioning tends to be weaker than that for forward or simultaneous conditioning. [**M. p33**]

10.4 **H.** Since humans seem more biologically prepared to develop phobias to small animals than some dangerous inanimate objects such as guns or cigarettes. [**B. p2**]

11. Concepts associated with Piaget

11.1 **B.** Feeling that all things have thoughts and emotions is termed 'animism' and is seen in the preoperational stage. [**B. p32**]

11.2 **F.** This probably best typifies egocentrism: children at the sensorimotor and preoperational stages of development tend to think that their way of perceiving a situation is the only way it can be perceived. [**L. p137–8**]

11.3 **H.** Before six months she would consider the rattle to have ceased to exist once it passed out of her field of perception. Such object permanence develops gradually until about eighteen months of age. [**B. p32**]

11.4 **G.** Development of knowledge of the laws of conservation is one of the achievements that marks the concrete operations stage. [**K. p51**]

12. Agnosias

12.1 **F, J.** Individuals with colour agnosia can tell differences between colours but not name them. Simultanagnosia refers to being able to perceive individual parts of a picture without being able to tell what the whole depicts. [**B. p20**]

12.2 **I.** This is the *mirror sign* and can occur in late Alzheimer's disease. [**K. p32**]

12.3   **E.** Autotopagnosia also refers to the inability to recognise or name body parts as well as point to them. **[B. p20]**

12.4   **B.** Anosognosia refers to the inability to recognise such deficits while anosodiaphoria refers to the lack of concern about the deficits that is sometimes seen following neurological insults. **[K. p32]**

13. Moral development

13.1   **A.** This is also known as the stage of moral relativism and this flexible attitude about moral issues occurs after the age of 10. **[L. p171–5]**

13.2   **B.** This is level 2 of his moral development theory. **[L. p176–80]**

13.3   **G.** She criticised Kohlberg for regarding the morality of justice as superior to the morality of care. **[L. p180–1]**

13.4   **I.** A review of this topic has shown that *induction* parenting style is more beneficial than love withdrawal or power assertion. **[L. p183–5]**

14. Theories of language development

14.1   **K.** Such speech is usually two-word utterances that leave out articles and prepositions. A single phrase can mean a number of different concepts at different times for the child. **[L. p155]**

14.2   **A.** Babbling is just one development of the prelinguistic stage, which lasts generally from birth to about one year of age. **[J. p279–280]**

14.3   **G.** Since he thinks this word refers to all such big animals. **[L. p154]**

14.4   **B.** This concept was proposed by Lenneberg and basically suggests that pre-pubertal children find it much easier to learn a new language than adolescents and adults. **[L. p158–9]**

15. Interpersonal attractiveness

15.1   **C.** Some researchers have found male attractiveness to be unrelated to dating frequency. **[Y. p650–4]**

15.2   **J.** Frequency of contact between the people concerned is the main reason for this. **[Y. p650–4]**

15.3   **D.** Over-disclosure gives rise to suspicion and reduces attraction. **[Y. p650–4]**

15.4   **F.** The primary drawback to being low in self-monitoring is a tendency to be unresponsive to the demands of different situations. **[Y. p650–4]**

16. Problem–solving and decision–making

16.1   **E.** His past experience of the questions leading up to the trick inhibit his problem-solving later. (In case it's late and you're suffering from study-fatigue, the answer should be that cattle drink water!) **[L. p400–2]**

16.2   **H.** An initial accidental learning of a fact leads to more coordinated responses in future. **[L. p397]**

16.3 **A.** A heuristic is a mental 'short-cut'. Media reports of terrorist activity tend to come to mind quickly, and so can distort one's judgement when estimating such a question. **[J. p300]**

16.4 **D.** This excellent fellow has come up with a novel way of using the presented materials (rather than being boring and poking the key out of the door onto the dishcloth and pulling it back into the room, or some such action) and is thus displaying De Bono's *lateral thinking*. **[J. p295]**

17. Learning theory

17.1 **C.** This procedure involves presenting the conditioned stimulus in the absence of an unconditioned stimulus. **[D. p413–18]**

17.2 **E.** These are more effective than imagined representations of the feared object. **[D. p413–18]**

17.3 **G.** Reinforcers that affect biological processes are known as primary reinforcers. **[D. p413–18]**

17.4 **H.** Joseph Wolpe pioneered this therapy. **[D. p413–18]**

18. Gender development

18.1 **C.** One of Freud's least developed and least popular theories. **[L. p194–5]**

18.2 **B.** The idea that gender remains stable over time is the next stage of development and occurs around the age of five or six years. **[L. p197]**

18.3 **A.** This was proposed by Bem. Degrees of masculinity and femininity can be assessed by the *Personal Attributes Questionnaire*. **[L. p199]**

18.4 **J.** It is important to be able to differentiate this from gender identity, which refers to the individual's concept of being male or female. **[L. p189]**

19. Goffman's theories of institutionalisation

19.1 **B.** This is the beginning step of the whole 'mortification process'. **[K. p65–6]**

19.2 **H.** The 'stripping' is both real and metaphorical to signify the individual's place in his new location. **[K. p65–6]**

19.3 **C.** There are elements of *batch living* here, but the patient's major resentment here relates to *binary living*: the way in which it appears that staff and inmates are inhabiting totally different worlds. **[B. p77–9]**

19.4 **E.** These changes can lead to what Barton termed *institutional neurosis*, which involves features such as withdrawal and submissiveness. **[B. p77–9]**

20. Visual perception

20.1 **J.** Somewhat convoluted, but the depiction has the components of two stationary objects at different distances from a moving observer. It is one of the monocular cues in depth perception. **[L. p362]**

20.2 **C.** Convergence also provides some indication of depth to the observer. Along with stereopsis and accommodation, it is a binocular cue. **[L. p362]**

20.3 **E.** This is one of the Gestalt laws of perception: minor gaps such as this are passed over and the figure is seen as a whole. **[K. p5]**

20.4 **L.** This is one of the concepts of object constancy in perception, and in this case, shape constancy is being demonstrated. **[B. p5]**

21. Behaviour modification

21.1 **F.** This involves exposure to a major fear-inducing situation. The situation can be real or contrived. **[D. p2114–17]**

21.2 **E.** Imagined scenes are embellished by the therapist and in successive approximation towards the patient's core fear. **[D. p2114–17]**

21.3 **I.** During the programmed practice the patients are on their own or with a safe person other than the therapist. **[D. p2114–17]**

22. Concepts of attachment

22.1 **E.** The mother *bonds* to her child, while the child becomes *attached* to its mother in due course. **[J. p463]**

22.2 **C.** Ainsworth's studies are important for the exam. Babies with anxious-avoidant attachment get upset at being left alone, not at their mothers' departures. Anxious-resistant attached babies do get upset when their mothers leave, but act in an ambivalent fashion to them when they return. **[J. p464–6]**

22.3 **I.** After about three months, babies enter the indiscriminate attachment stage, in which they start to show preferences for familiar people, but are still relatively happy with strangers. The social smile seen in the pre-attachment period tends to fade over this later period. **[J. p460]**

22.4 **B.** This refers to our social interactions: anxious individuals tend to have a greater need for affiliation to help them get through a tough period. **[L. p211–12]**

23. Theory of emotion

23.1 **E.** The emotional feelings come from awareness of such arousal. **[Y. p430–3]**

23.2 **D.** The perception first activates the thalamus, which in turn alerts both the cortex and the hypothalamus for action. **[Y. p430–3]**

23.3 **F.** Specific emotions are assumed to result from various appraisals, such as an appraisal of threat leading to anxiety. **[Y. p430–3]**

23.4 **B.** There is experimental support to this theory. **[Y. p430–3]**

24. Personality assessment

24.1 **B.** It is in a true/false format and is not recommended for purposes other than as a screening device. **[D. p705–10]**

24.2 **I.** It has sixteen personality dimensions and has limited usefulness with clinical populations. **[D. p705–10]**

24.3 **J.** A widely used method, it is time consuming and needs training to interpret responses. **[D. p705–10]**

24.4 **H.** It is administered briefly and can be adjusted to clinical interviews. **[D. p705–10]**

25. Prejudice

25.1 **A.** The Milgram experiments support this concept. However, the emphasis on individual differences does not explain prejudice in all situations. **[L. p223–9]**

25.2 **E.** Runciman's relative deprivation theory does not explain the processes involved in producing fraternalistic deprivation. **[L. p223–9]**

25.3 **B.** According to Allport, increased contact between prejudiced individuals reduces prejudice. **[L. p223–9]**

25.4 **G.** This is true when the people competing do not know each other for a long time. **[L. p223–9]**

26. Stages of development

26.1 **D.** This is object permanence and develops during Piaget's sensori-motor stage (0-2 years). **[L. p136]**

26.2 **B.** It is important to know the normal range of milestones such as this, particularly for the clinical exams. Candidates are sometimes disconcerted to be asked to state these ranges when they report in the history 'milestones were normal'. **[D. p655]**

26.3 **A.** 18 to 30 months is the general time given for the two-word sentence period. **[J. p281]**

26.4 **F.** Twelve-year-olds should be able to do this, but you were not told how long she is able to perform this in the stem. **[J. p596]**

27. Self–concept and growth

27.1 **C.** Self-efficacy belief is associated with career development and health-related behaviour. **[R. p391–430]**

27.2 **I.** Reinterpretation gives new understanding to that person. **[R. p391–430]**

27.3 **D.** Growth motivation excites further, whereas deficit motivation does not create more needs. **[R. p391–430]**

27.4 **H.** Positive regard can be conditional and unconditional. Conditions of worth are evidenced by conditional positive and negative regards. **[R. p391–430]**

28. Prosocial behaviour

28.1 **C.** One person witnessing the event tends to act more readily since he bears the social responsibility alone; in the group, this responsibility is spread around, so that individuals feel less pressure to act. **[L. p247–8]**

28.2 **G.** The students are looking for hints from others that they should react, but many of these others are looking at them for the same reason. This can lead to a collective inactivity among many of the group. **[J. p435]**

28.3   **F.** On the other hand, the empathy–altruism hypothesis
highlights the role of empathetic leanings: the negative-state
relief model is a modification of this hypothesis. **[L. p243–4]**

28.4   **B.** It is hypothesised to be an in-built form of prosocial behaviour
and is seen in many species. Psychological altruism, however, is
confined to humans. **[J. p442]**

29. Theories of moral development

29.1   **F.** This is also known as heteronomous morality. It is the middle
stage of Piaget's three stages of moral development, the other two
being the premoral period and the stage of moral relativism. **[L.
p174]**

29.2   **B.** This is stage four of Kohlberg's six stages and is part of his
second level of conventional morality. **[L. p177]**

29.3   **C.** This is Kohlberg's final stage of moral development and forms
part of his postconventional morality. Few act at this level for the
majority of their actions, with the exception, for example, of
individuals generally thought of as saints. **[B. p34]**

29.4   **D.** According to her, males tend to focus on rules and principles
and thus display a morality of justice. **[L. p180]**

30. Perception and cognition

30.1   **J.** Pigeonholing refers to reducing perceptual information needed
to place a specific stimulus into a specific category. **[D. p386–9]**

30.2   **A.** Hence patients may be able to recall indirectly and be
influenced by events and stimuli that they cannot recall having
perceived consciously. **[D. p386–9]**

30.3   **G.** As implicit memory is behavioural, emotional and perceptual.
[D. p386–9]

30.4   **I.** Unlike serial process, the parallel process can function
simultaneously with numerous other functions without inhibiting
them. **[D. p386–9]**

31. Psychological testing

31.1   **G, I.** This EMI is made more difficult by not specifying how
many answers you should select: you will certainly be told how
many you have to choose in the exam. Projective personality tests
are unstructured and generally involve the patient interpreting
an ambiguous picture or storyline. The MMPI is an objective
personality test that presents many statements that those tested
have to answer as true or false. Note that these tests may be of
dubious benefit if the patient has an organic condition. **[D.
p704–12]**

31.2   **B.** Simple but useful: this should be a routine part of your
cognitive assessment in the mental state examination.
Increasingly longer sequences of numbers are spoken to the
patient: he is then asked to repeat these. The patient is tested in
his ability both to recount numbers forwards, then to recount
numbers backwards. **[D. p698]**

31.3   **E.** Since this is an 'over-learned' skill and would be less prone to being affected by an organic brain syndrome. This test is of limited use, however, if the patient has a history of dyslexia. **[E. p99]**

31.4   **H, J.** The patient must be suspected of having a frontal-lobe syndrome, therefore tests of executive functioning should be performed. Other such tests include verbal fluency, the Luria, and the Card Sorting Test. **[E. p98]**

32. Behaviour theory

32.1   **F.** The Premack principle is particularly useful when it is difficult to identify reinforcers. **[R. p364–72]**

32.2   **G.** This is the behaviour she enjoys doing most of the time. **[R. p364–72]**

32.3   **E.** The response is reinforced here. **[R. p364–72]**

32.4   **C.** It does not matter whether the high probability behaviour is pleasurable or not: the probability of indulging in this behaviour should be high. This question is basically the standard single-item question of the rest of the paper: the contrasts in strategies in answering the traditional MCQs and the EMIs are evident. **[R. p364–72]**

33. Behaviour therapy

33.1   **H.** This mechanism involves changing the magnitude of the unconditional response. **[D. p2083–5]**

33.2   **G.** The social situation regularly follows certain behaviours. This is contrast to reinforcement with, for example, earning points for artwork, which would be a contrived reinforcer. **[D. p2083–5]**

33.3   **D.** The conditioned response is modified by replacing the unconditioned stimulus (UCS) with another UCS that elicits an unconditioned response (UCR) that is incompatible with that of the original one. **[D. p2083–5]**

33.4   **F.** When the individual is pre-exposed to a neutral stimulus in the absence of the UCS, a response develops less readily to this stimulus. **[D. p2083–5]**

34. Concepts of forgetting

34.1   **A.** This is a form of cue-dependent forgetting: context-dependent forgetting describes difficulties in recall without external cues that were present when the material was learned. Note that, while answer B is an appropriate answer for this question, EMIs demand that you select the *most* appropriate answer. **[J. p262]**

34.2   **F.** This term is referring to repression: the individual is motivated to forget portions of their experiences that are laden with negative emotions. **[L. p389; J. p264]**

34.3   **G.** Since the man's previous learning of driving in a car with a right-sided steering wheel is interfering with his learning how to drive one with a left-sided steering wheel. **[J. p263]**

34.4   **J.** This is another form of cue-dependent forgetting: state-dependent forgetting. The internal cue of the anxiety provoked by the situation helps him to remember things he forgets when relaxed. **[J. p262]**

35. Behavioural analysis

35.1   **G.** This is an altering response reflexively elicited by the new stimulus to direct the dog's attention to the unconditional stimulus. **[D. p2080–1]**
35.2   **I.** The bell (CS) signals the imminent presentation of food (UCS). **[D. p2080–1]**
35.3   **J.** The food (UCS) elicits a definite response (salivation). **[D. p2080–1]**
35.4   **A.** The dog is receiving food (UCS) because of the bell (CS), not because of salivating (UCR). **[D. p2080–1]**

36. Theories and concepts of emotion

36.1   **H.** The James-Lange theory suggests that physical behaviour and sensations feedback are responsible for setting up the emotional response: in this case, the arousal caused by having to go into flight mode causes the anxiety. **[L. p81–3]**
36.2   **C.** Lazarus' suggestion was that our emotional response is largely dependent on how we interpret the meaning and context of a given stimulus. **[L. p87–9]**
36.3   **E.** This hypothesis is a specific form of the James-Lange theory. **[J. p136]**
36.4   **J.** A curious term proposed by LeDoux: the amygdala is proposed as a seat for emotional memory. **[D. p449]**

37. Neurodevelopment

37.1   **D.** The assessment of sequential appearance of prelinguistic vocalisations is important in the early diagnosis of developmental disabilities. **[Q. p6–12]**
37.2   **A.** The test results correlate with intellectual ability, learning disorders and psychological disturbances. **[Q. p6–12]**
37.3   **F.** As several factors interfere with motor performance. **[Q. p6–12]**
37.4   **H.** Social milestones are communicative in origin. **[Q. p6–12]**

38. Social influence

38.1   **L.** While some aspects of this are reminiscent of autocratic leadership, this is more descriptive of Fiedler's *contingency theory*. Task-oriented leadership is contrasted with relationship-oriented leadership. Individuals are classified by how they respond to questions about how they view their *least preferred co-worker*. **[K. p23]**
38.2   **J.** This shares some characteristics of groupthink and diffusion of responsibility, but the combination of convincing each other that nothing is wrong and that no one is to blame is typical of pluralistic ignorance. **[M. p32–3]**

38.3 **F.** This individual is enjoying some social power by virtue of her expertise in this area. **[B. p15]**

38.4 **A.** The *co-action effect* refers to improved performance on a task when others around are doing the same task. Along with the audience effect, these are examples of *social facilitation*. **[L. p255–6]**

Psychopharmacology EMIs

39. Physical emergencies during antipsychotic treatment
39.1 **G.** Use of high potency antipsychotics, high dose treatment, initiation of treatment and dose titration are the times of increased risk for NMS. **[T. p93–4]**
39.2 **B.** CPK is increased due to myolysis. **[T. p93–4]**
39.3 **C.** In the future an antipsychotic from a different group may be re-challenged using very small doses. **[T. p93–4]**
39.4 **L.** 20–30%. **[T. p93–4]**

40. Extrapyramidal side–effects
40.1 **L.** These adverse events most commonly occur during this period. **[T. p93–5]**
40.2 **E.** This is the only EPS that responds fully to anticholinergic treatment. **[T. p93–5]**
40.3 **F.** High CPK levels are a striking finding in neuroleptic malignant syndrome. **[T. p93–5]**
40.4 **D.** The tremor of idiopathic Parkinsonism is less common and tends to occur later in treatment, if at all. **[T. p93–5]**

41. Antipsychotics
41.1 **D.** Olanzapine is currently the only drug available of the thienobenzodiazepine class. **[T. p82–5]**
41.2 **F.** Other dibenzothiazepines are metiapine and clothiapine. **[T. p82–5]**
41.3 **H.** Since it has low EPS when used in low doses, it is considered an 'atypical' antipsychotic by some. **[T. p82–5]**
41.4 **E.** This property may have clinical applications for patients who are intermittently compliant with medication. **[T. p82–5]**

42. Pharmacokinetics
42.1 **B.** As the clearance mechanism is not saturated, drug clearance is a linear function of that drug's blood concentration. **[T. p46]**
42.2 **D.** No linear relationship exists between the drug's blood concentration and its clearance. **[T. p46]**
42.3 **D.** As in 42.2 above. **[T. p46]**
42.4 **B.** As in 42.1 above. **[T. p46]**

43. Early side–effects of antipsychotic treatment
43.1 **A.** 90% of them occur within days of exposure or dose increase. **[T. p93–5]**
43.2 **G.** This involuntary action involves the tongue sweeping the inner buccal surface. **[T. p93–5]**

43.3 **B.** 40% of the patients who are on typical antipsychotics develop this over a two-week period. The incidence is very low with clozapine. **[T. p93–5]**

44. Mood stabilisers

44.1 **A.** Hence it may warrant dose titration for the first three months. **[T. p124–9]**

44.2 **H.** It also displaces carbamazepine from protein-binding sites and thus can result in transient toxicity. **[T. p124–9]**

44.3 **F.** White blood counts may be increased by 40% commonly in the first week of lithium exposure. **[T. p124–9]**

44.4 **H.** Valproate can also rarely cause hepatotoxicity and Stevens-Johnson syndrome. **[T. p124–9]**

45. Adverse effects of the atypical antipsychotics

45.1 **A, F.** While the potential for risperidone to cause extrapyramidal side-effects (EPSE) is well recognised, especially at higher doses, amisulpride may also cause them. Overall, however, the incidence of EPSE with both drugs is low in comparison to most of the typical antipsychotics. **[H. p87]**

45.2 **G.** Clozapine and sertindole are associated with the most postural hypotension from the above, but the former is obviously ruled out by the stem. **[H. p87]**

45.3 **C.** Clozapine has the most sedation of the above, followed by olanzapine and quetiapine. **[H. p87]**

46. Antidepressant–related receptor and amine changes

46.1 **H.** MAOIs may also have this effect. **[T. p73]**

46.2 **B.** This difference in action from antidepressants may be a reason why some patients with medication-resistant depression respond to ECT. **[T. p72–3]**

46.3 **G.** Noradrenaline and dopamine are other monoamines broken down by MAO. **[T. p72–3]**

46.4 **J.** Amphetamine and fenfluramine also have this action. **[T. p72–3]**

47. Anxiolytics and hypnotics

47.1 **A.** It is unlikely that you will get many EMIs of this type. Part of the attraction of EMIs is that clinical vignettes, for example, can be given and candidates are thus forced to synthesise the information to see which elements are essential for answering. This question, however, is not examining such higher functioning: it is merely seeing if you can remember snippets of pharmacokinetics and pharmacodynamics. To get back to this answer: buspirone also has antagonistic activity at dopamine D_2 receptors. **[G. p364]**

47.2 **H.** The agent in the list of options least likely to cause a hangover effect is zaleplon, as it has an elimination half-life of only one hour. **[G. p365]**

47.3   **C.** Even if you could not remember that diazepam is metabolised
to oxazepam, this would still be very 'guessable' as diazepam has
the longest half-life by far of the three listed benzodiazepines.
[G. p360]

47.4   **E.** Paraldehyde best fits this bill: both of these facts are explained
by its characteristic excretion via the lungs. **[G. p367]**

48. Adverse effects of typical antipsychotics

48.1   **H.** However, hyperprolactinaemia is responsible for breast
engorgement and galactorrhoea. **[T. p87–96]**

48.2   **B.** Chlorpromazine is commonly associated with these changes.
[T. p87–96]

48.3   **D.** Increased synchronisation and increased slow-wave activity
come with long-term antipsychotic treament. **[T. p93]**

48.4   **C.** It need not be very hot for such patients to suffer severe
burns. **[T. p92]**

49. Psychotropic use in lactating mothers

49.1   **J.** From case reports, citalopram was associated with uneasy sleep
in an infant and fluoxetine use caused adverse effects in two
infants. **[H. p211–15]**

49.2   **C.** Doxepin caused reversible adverse effects in two infants. **[H.
p211–15]**

49.3   **K.** Some studies reported lethargy in infants whose mothers were
on chlorpromazine. **[H. p211–15]**

49.4   **H.** Long-acting benzodiazepines cause lethargy, sedation and
weight loss in infants. **[H. p211–15]**

50. Pharmacological profiles of the newer antidepressants

50.1   **E.** Its metabolism is mediated via several cytochrome P450
enzymes, which generally means it is less likely to be affected by
the effects of concomitant medications. **[T. p110–5]**

50.2   **F.** It is highly protein bound and acts selectively on the
noradrenergic system. **[T. p110–5]**

50.3   **D.** Though the findings are controversial, some case reports have
suggested the strong possibility of blood dyscrasia with this agent.
[T. p110–5]

51. Pharmacokinetics terms

51.1   **G.** No gold stars for this one: oral administration of morphine
leads to significant hepatic metabolism when absorbed drug is
transported there via the portal system. **[D. p2250–2]**

51.2   **J.** Since saturation of the enzymes responsible for its metabolism
occurs. Phenytoin is another drug that shows zero-order kinetics
in elimination. **[D. p2250–2]**

51.3   **B.** Chlorpromazine has a relatively low bioavailability fraction of
10–33%. **[D. p2361]**

51.4   **D.** Levo-dopa, but not dopamine, can cross the blood–brain
barrier. **[B. p163]**

52. Commencing clozapine treatment

52.1   **E.** If this occurs it is generally a problem in the first month of treatment; it occasionally persists, however. **[H. p50]**

52.2   **C, D.** Pyrexia is quite frequent in the first three weeks and should not lead by itself to cessation of therapy. **[H. p50]**

52.3   **H.** While one could select a number of appropriate options for this stem, the one crucial choice is that you should now consider a referral to cardiology, as there is the possibility of a clozapine-induced myocarditis (although this is rare). Fever and chest pain are other suggestive features of this. **[H. p50]**

52.4   **A, I.** Relatively straightforward in this situation: quit medicine immediately if you chose 'J' for this stem. **[H. p50]**

53. Adverse effects of antidepressants

53.1   **H.** An easy one to start you off: MAOIs can interact with sympathomimetics and this reinforces the importance of discussing prohibited over-the-counter preparations with patients. **[F. p633]**

53.2   **E.** While this question allows you to cut down the list of options to just three, you still have to know that fluoxetine is the agent most likely to cause headache and reduced appetite. **[G. p260]**

53.3   **A.** Dothiepin, however, is higher on the fatal toxicity index of antidepressants than amitriptyline. **[G. p245]**

53.4   **A.** Dothiepin and mianserin are also antidepressants with marked sedative effects. **[I. p136]**

54. Pharmacology of pregnancy and the puerperium

54.1   **H.** Trifluoperazine and chlorpromazine are the agents whose use has been most reported in pregnancy. Both olanzapine and clozapine appear to be relatively safe, but experience with their use is more limited. **[H. p209]**

54.2   **A.** While most experience is with tricyclics such as nortriptyline, amitriptyline and imipramine, there is a reasonable amount of experience suggesting that fluoxetine is relatively safe. **[H. p206–9]**

54.3   **F.** While both paroxetine and sertraline are excreted into breast milk, infant serum levels of these drugs have been shown to be very low, and so they are probably safe to give to the breast-feeding mother. Infant serum levels of fluoxetine tend to be a little higher in this situation. **[H. p211–12]**

54.4   **I.** Zolpidem is to be preferred over zopiclone as there is more evidence to suggest that excreted amounts are minimal with no observed effects on nursed infants. **[H. p211, 214]**

55. Choice of antidepressants

55.1   **J.** Due to its amphetamine-like structure. **[H. p110–15]**

55.2   **E.** It may also alter insulin requirements. **[H. p110–15]**

55.3   **D.** Citalopram and sertraline also have active metabolites with weak action. **[H. p110–15]**

55.4 **H.** It is also licensed for depression, OCD, PTSD, social phobia and panic disorder. **[H. p110–15]**

56. Drugs of use in substance misuse treatment

56.1 **A.** The main strategy in answering EMIs is to use the given information to whittle away options from the list. This gentleman has alcohol dependence so options B, D, H, I and J can be safely discarded. The actual side-effects listed could be caused by either of the benzodiazepines, acamprosate or disulfiram, according to the BNF, so we need to use other information to be able to select the most likely agent. We are told that he is commenced on this agent for his dependence, rather than any co-morbid problems, and that he has already had detoxification, so this reduces the options to A and G. He continues to abuse alcohol, but only reports relatively mild side-effects, so this effectively rules out G. In this way you can reduce a large list of options to just a few, from which we may judge the most appropriate answer. **[F. p246–7]**

56.2 **G.** This woman has suffered an alcohol-disulfiram reaction leading to the build-up of acetaldehyde in her plasma. It is important to warn patients about such less obvious sources of alcohol such as elixirs and some prepared foods. **[G. p375–6]**

56.3 **D.** This is Raynaud's phenomenon, and clonidine is the agent most likely to cause this. Lofexidine has similar actions to clonidine, but causes less hypotension. **[F. p87; G. p373–4]**

57. Effects of antidepressants on receptors

57.1 **A.** Postural hypotension, drowsiness and ejaculatory failure are the main effects of α_1-adrenoreceptor blockade. **[B. p167]**

57.2 **B.** Histamine H_1-receptor blockade can also cause weight gain. **[W. p33–7]**

57.3 **E.** As in 57.2 above. **[W. p33–7]**

57.4 **C.** While drugs with serotonergic and dopaminergic effects can have adverse effects on sexual functioning, the effects via dopamine are indirect: the rise in prolactin causes the sexual difficulties. **[B. p166–7, P. p550]**

58. Pharmacokinetics and pharmacodynamics of the benzodiazepines

58.1 **E.** The opening of the chloride channels by GABA stimulation is achieved by allosteric modulation. **[T. p131–7]**

58.2 **I.** This is because diazepam distributes rapidly and thus its plasma concentration falls rapidly. **[T. p131–7]**

58.3 **B.** A study showed that it was only events after the drug was given that were forgotten. **[T. p131–7]**

59. Side–effects of antidepressants

59.1 **H.** One of the difficulties with EMIs is that frequently a number of the options can 'fit' a given stem: the candidate is generally asked to select the option that is most likely to be correct, which inevitably calls for careful judgement. While many antidepressants can cause a lowering of the seizure threshold, maprotiline is the drug most likely to do this from the options, especially in higher doses. **[I. p136; F. p191]**

59.2 **A.** Among the most sedative of the antidepressants are amitriptyline, dothiepin and mianserin. **[I. p136]**

59.3 **E.** Again a common side-effect; however, fluvoxamine is particularly associated with severe nausea in some patients. Remember 'v' is for 'vomit'! **[I. p196]**

59.4 **K.** The MAOIs are associated with peripheral neuritis/neuropathy and paraesthesia. It is thought that these may be a result of pyridoxine deficiency. **[F. p192–3]**

60. Pharmacodynamics of anxiolytic medications

60.1 **G.** She is displaying activity indicative of benzodiazepine dependence. Lorazepam has the highest dependence potential of these agents, a function of its very short half-life. **[I. p135]**

60.2 **D, F, G.** These three cause the most marked sedative effects. Buspirone is the least sedating, followed by propranolol and clobazam. **[I. p135]**

60.3 **G.** If a benzodiazepine must be used in patients with hepatic impairment, those with short half-lives and fewest active metabolites are best: both lorazepam and oxazepam fulfil these criteria. **[H. p228]**

60.4 **C.** Although this is a rare effect of buspirone, it is the most likely of the listed agents to cause tachycardia. **[F. p172]**

61. Lithium

61.1 **G.** About 70% is absorbed here, while 20% is absorbed in the stomach. **[T. p120]**

61.2 **G.** Same answer, since this is the site of maximal absorption; this process is speeded when concentrations are high since the process is one of passive diffusion. **[T. p120]**

61.3 **H.** The absorption of lithium in the stomach does not appear to be affected by the ambient pH. **[T. p120]**

61.4 **A.** Doses split three times daily do this: a single nighttime dose can give up to a fourfold difference. **[T. p121]**

62. Pharmacodynamics of hypnotic agents

62.1 **E.** He is likely to be dependent on the agent; temazepam is the agent above most likely to cause dependence. **[I. p134]**

62.2 **A.** The chloral derivatives tend to be associated with marked gastrointestinal effects in a number of patients. **[I. p134]**

62.3 **C.** The hangover effect is related to its long half-life: up to 36 hours in this age group, and even longer in the elderly. Flunitrazepam causes somewhat less of such an effect. **[I. p134]**

62.4   **H.** Hallucinations have also been associated with zopiclone therapy. **[F. p168]**

63. Antidepressants: adverse effects

63.1   **J.** This may be the reason for trazodone's ability to cause priapism. **[T. p113–17]**

63.2   **H.** This is the most common adverse effect of SSRIs (25–35%). **[T. p113–17]**

63.3   **F.** Due to their quinidine-like actions. **[T. p113–17]**

63.4   **G.** Due to its long half-life. **[T. p113–17]**

64. Anticholinergic drugs

64.1   **A.** You should suspect anticholinergic abuse in this man. While many drugs in this class can give users a high if abused, procyclidine and benzhexol have the greatest abuse potential. Of the two, benzhexol has the greater stimulant activity. **[G. p304–5]**

64.2   **E.** Recent research has noted the high toxicity of orphenadrine and deaths have occurred with large overdoses. **[G. p305]**

64.3   **H.** MAOIs are contraindicated because of this risk: tetrabenazine causes the release of amines in a similar fashion to reserpine. **[G. p306]**

65. Anticonvulsant agents

65.1   **E.** Lamotrigine is a promising agent in the treatment of bipolar depression. However, up to 10% of patents develop a rash, which means treatment must be stopped, as a proportion will progress to Stevens-Johnson syndrome. Rash and headache are also found with carbamazepine treatment, but the rash is less frequent (around 10% versus 3%). **[K. p185]**

65.2   **I.** Topiramate has the unique effect of causing weight loss among patients on this class of drugs. It inhibits carbonic anhydrase and also holds promise for the treatment of bipolar disorder. **[G. p350–1]**

65.3   **J.** A number of anticonvulsants can cause psychotic or depressive symptoms. Vigabatrin, however, has been the only such agent to be associated with an irreversible reduction of peripheral vision and thus requires visual field monitoring during treatment. **[G. p351]**

65.4   **F.** Phenobarbitone has also been associated with osteoporosis, rashes and cognitive impairment and is thus no longer first-line treatment for epilepsy. **[K. p184]**

66. Pharmacodynamics of antidepressants

66.1   **D, H, L.** The effects of venlafaxine on monoamine reuptake are dose-related: serotonin reuptake inhibition alone occurs at low doses, while dopamine reuptake inhibition only occurs at high doses. **[W. p62]**

66.2 **B, F, I, J.** Mirtazapine allows the selective stimulation of the postsynaptic $5HT_{1a}$ subclass of serotonergic receptors by antagonising both $5HT_2$ and $5HT_3$ subclasses. This allows the drug to have clinical efficacy but with reduced serotonergic side-effects such as nausea, sexual dysfunction or agitation. **[W. p70]**

66.3 **H, I, L.** The term 'selective serotonin reuptake inhibitor' is relative. Fluoxetine has weaker effect at noradrenaline reuptake inhibition and can agonise $5HT_{2C}$ receptors to a degree. **[P. p235]**

66.4 **D, H.** Bupropion is used mainly in Great Britain and Ireland as an aid to smoking cessation. It is associated with a higher rate of seizures than most other antidepressants, and has been suggested anecdotally to be less likely to cause 'switching' into hypomania than other antidepressants. **[W. p80–1]**

67. Pharmacodynamics of anti–manic agents

67.1 **E.** Because of its small size, lithium can interact with many electrolyte channels. **[G. p331]**

67.2 **I.** Glutamate inhibition and/or GABA potentiation are common to anticonvulsants. **[P. p270–2]**

67.3 **E.** These are also thought to be important modes of action of lithium. It is crucial to read the instructions about whether you may use the same response more than once, if such instructions are given. **[G. p331]**

68. Impairment of glucose tolerance and atypical antipsychotics

68.1 **C.** Such patients need not have a positive family history of diabetes. **[H. p80–2]**

68.2 **D.** It is thought that olanzapine has more potential to cause diabetes than typical antipsychotics or risperidone. **[H. p80–2]**

68.3 **E.** This is a curious suggestion, since quetiapine therapy is associated with an increased risk of developing diabetes itself. **[H. p80–2]**

69. Drug interactions

69.1 **E, H.** While alcohol can obviously cause such a tyramine crisis, gin is somewhat less likely to do this. Other drugs that can precipitate this reaction include cocaine, barbiturates and L-Dopa. **[K. p178]**

69.2 **D, I.** It is essential to know the list of agents that can precipitate lithium toxicity both for exam purposes and to keep you out of the courts. Frusemide and amiloride are relatively safe with lithium. Non-steroidal anti-inflammatory agents and thiazide diuretics still account for most of such reactions. **[G. p335]**

69.3 **C, G.** Paraldehyde's metabolism is blocked by disulfiram and can lead to a build-up of acetaldehyde. Benzodiazepines can also interact with its metabolism but do not cause the reaction. **[G. p377]**

69.4 **C, G.** The same two answers: this time methadone acts to potentiate the central nervous system depressant effects of the alcohol and paraldehyde. **[G. p368–9]**

70. Monoamine oxidase inhibitors

70.1   **A.** Supine hypotension is more common with MAOI treatment than with tricyclic antidepressant treatment. **[T. p108–10]**

70.2   **F.** It builds up over the first four weeks of exposure to the agents. **[T. p108–10]**

70.3   **I.** Tranylcypromine can precipitate an encephalopathy-type picture. **[T. p108–10]**

70.4   **E.** Because of its very high tyramine content. **[T. p108–10]**

71. Drugs in dementia

71.1   **D.** Other antioxidants tried have been vitamins C and E. *Ginkgo biloba* is thought to cause a degree of cognitive enhancement. **[G. p353]**

71.2   **F.** Other such drugs have been found equally ineffective: papavarine, anticoagulants and carbonic anhydrase inhibitors, among others. **[P. p490]**

71.3   **A, E.** Both of these act as precursors for acetylcholine synthesis: lecithin is phosphatidyl choline. **[G. p356]**

71.4   **B, C, G, H.** Most of the cholinesterase inhibitors in use are relatively selective for acetylcholinesterase. Tacrine and metrifonate have some efficacy and inhibit pseudocholinesterase as well. **[P. p467, 481–3]**

72. Side-effects of the newer antidepressants

72.1   **J, G.** Unsurprisingly, nausea is the most common side-effect, occurring with an incidence above that of placebo of some 10% to 30%. A fine tremor is found in 10% above placebo levels (all subsequent percentages in these answers are those occurring above placebo levels). **[G. p259]**

72.2   **F, I, B.** Reboxetine causes excess stimulation of the sympathetic nervous system over the parasympathetic nervous system, thus giving some symptoms similar to those of the tricyclic antidepressants. Dry mouth occurs in 11%, while insomnia and constipation each occur at a 9% incidence. **[G. p270]**

72.3   **J, E.** Nausea is common (25%) with venlafaxine, as is drowsiness (14%). **[G. p271]**

72.4   **E, F, L.** Drowsiness is the most common with 9–14% of patients reporting this above placebo, followed by dry mouth and increased appetite or weight gain, each occurring in about 9%. **[G. p273]**

73. Side-effects of antipsychotics

73.1   **B.** The most striking features are the sedation and the anticholinergic side-effects, with some extrapyramidal side-effects (EPSE). **[I. p138]**

73.2   **G.** From the combination of cardiac effects, EPSE and low sedation. **[I. p138]**

73.3   **C.** There is marked sedation, as well as anticholinergic effects and weight gain. **[I. p138]**

74. *Signs of lithium toxicity.*

74.1 **C, E, G.** Occasionally an EMI can instruct you that you can use a given option only once as an answer, as in this question. In effect, this question is asking you to rank these symptoms in terms of their appearance as lithium toxicity progresses. Toxicity need not be present for these three side-effects to occur. **[G. p331–5]**

74.2 **H, I.** Other signs of mild lithium toxicity include nausea and diarrhoea, but the latter has been used for the first part already. **[G. p334]**

74.3 **B, D, J, L.** Drowsiness and cerebellar ataxia may also become apparent at this stage. **[G. p334]**

74.4 **A, F, K.** This is generally associated with levels around and above 2 mmol/l and is an obvious emergency. The deterioration in mental state begun in the last two stages worsens and can result in coma and death. **[G. p334, K. p180]**

Descriptive and Psychodynamic Psychopathology EMIs

75. Defence mechanisms
75.1 **K.** Since it is a conscious decision to exclude such thoughts, *suppression* rather than *repression* is being employed here. **[O. p755–7]**
75.2 **L.** Undoing relates to actions or utterances that are designed to counteract unacceptable ideas. Along with isolation and repression, it is seen in many patients with obsessive-compulsive disorder. **[O. p755–7]**
75.3 **G.** Rationalisation involves blaming an external subject or event for one's own unacceptable thoughts or actions. Along with denial, it is one of the main defence mechanisms seen in individuals with substance misuse. **[D. p584–5]**
75.4 **J.** Thereby allowing an outlet of unacceptable desires in a way accepted by society. Sublimation and humour are considered mature defence mechanisms. **[D. p584–5]**

76. Individuals associated with psychopathological syndromes
76.1 **G.** An easy one to start you off. These associations tend to come up mainly on the individual statements questions. You should know these thoroughly as they can act as references *in extremis* for the MRCPsych part II essay. The quoted reference has some such lists that, while not exhaustive, are a very useful start for memorising. **[K. p243–4]**
76.2 **F.** It was described first by him in 1873. **[A. p336]**
76.3 **J.** He described it as a reduction in 'nervous energy'. **[M. p69]**
76.4 **D.** Gull is only one of the first to describe systematically anorexia nervosa: others include Lasègue and Marcé. Gull has also been proposed by some crime writers as having been Jack the Ripper in his spare time. It's important to have interests outside of medicine. **[M. p80]**

77. Psychopathological syndromes
77.1 **H.** This is the Frégoli delusion in which the patient is usually persecuted by an individual, and only the patient recognises the individual through his/her disguise. Both Frégoli syndrome and Capgras' syndrome are examples of misidentification syndromes in which various difficulties in face recognition pathways have been proposed. **[A. p118–20]**

77.2 **D.** Cotard's syndrome is associated with the features of severe depression with psychotic features in older patients. Nihilistic delusions are among the most striking of these and, if prominent, suggest very severe depression. **[A. p122]**

77.3 **J.** Meadow was the first to describe Munchausen's by proxy: it is also known as Polle's syndrome. Briquet's syndrome on the other hand refers to an established pattern of multiple physical complaints in a number of systems in the presenting patient that remain medically unexplained (somatisation disorder). **[A. p221]**

77.4 **E.** It is part of the definition of the Couvade syndrome that it is not a delusion belief. Instead, the husband (and rarely other family members) can develop to a greater or lesser degree some of the physical symptoms associated with pregnancy. It is most marked in the third and ninth months of the pregnancy. **[A. p261]**

78. Disturbance of mood

78.1 **F.** According to Snaith and Taylor, outwardly expressed irritability is an independent mood disorder on its own, independent of anxiety, depression and other mood states. **[A. p306–7]**

78.2 **K.** On the other hand, inwardly directed irritability is common in obsessive compulsive disorder. **[A. p306–7]**

78.3 **E.** In other words, the severity of irritability is generally greater, the younger the patient. **[A. p306–7]**

78.4 **D.** The irritable individual always experiences this state as unpleasant. **[A. p306–7]**

79. Employment of defence mechanisms

79.1 **B.** The defence mechanisms are another area of the curriculum that lends itself well to generating lists: expect to see many EMIs on this area over coming sittings of the exam. **[U. p29]**

79.2 **G.** He is in luck: the limit on the number of allowed attempts has been lifted recently. He is using 'sour grapes' to cope with his distress. **[U. p27]**

79.3 **F.** He projects his repressed impulse onto her. **[U. p26–7]**

79.4 **I.** Regression is adaptive at times: activities on holiday are an example. **[U. p29–30]**

80. Delusional beliefs

80.1 **F.** De Clérambault's syndrome is just one form of erotomania: the recipient of the attentions in erotomania need not be of a higher social status. It is more common in females and can be a mood-congruent delusion in manic episodes. **[A. p117–18]**

80.2 **A.** The Capgras' syndrome is also known as *l'illusion de sosies* and is one of the delusional misidentification syndromes. **[B. p88]**

80.3 **H.** Cotard's syndrome generally signifies a severe depressive episode and the delusions are usually bizarre in nature. **[A. p121–2]**

80.4   **G.** This is a passivity phenomenon and is one of Schneider's first-rank symptoms of schizophrenia. **[B. p89]**

81. Disorders of movement and behaviour
81.1   **A.** Hyperactivity is a description of behaviour rather than a subjective sense of current state. **[A. p334–5]**
81.2   **E.** This is the motor equivalent of thought block in the flow of speech. **[A. p337]**
81.3   **G.** This is a particular form of grimacing. **[A. p337]**
81.4   **D.** He is doing the opposite of what is expected of him (that is, facing the examiner). **[A. p336–7]**

82. Psychopathological features of severe depression
82.1   **C.** These symptoms are of concern as they may be associated with the patient attempting suicide. **[A. p121]**
82.2   **I.** It is important to remember the eponym for such symptoms, *Cotard's syndrome*, as this tends to be a favourite among examiners. **[A. p121–2]**
82.3   **J.** As it worsens this can become depressive stupor. **[B. p83]**
82.4   **E.** Patients tend to find it very difficult to describe depersonalisation or derealisation. The patient is not delusional: he describes his experience as an 'as if' situation. These phenomena also occur in less severe forms of depression and can also occur in the healthy individual when fatigued. **[A. p203–7]**

83. Bipolar affective disorder and perceptual abnormalities
83.1   **J.** This is a recognised feature of elation. **[T. p256–8]**
83.2   **E.** The illusion occurring at a time of mood disturbance is termed an *affect illusion*. **[T. p256–8]**
83.3   **D.** This is not a complex experience, as, for example, are music or voices. **[T. p256–8]**
83.4   **B, I.** This is a mood-congruent hallucination. **[T. p256–8]**

84. Psychopathological features of anxiety–related states
84.1   **J.** Simple phobias are examples of situational anxiety: the anxiety only arises when certain situations are encountered. **[A. p302]**
84.2   **E.** There is no specific precipitant for the anxiety as in situational anxiety. **[B. p86]**
84.3   **G.** This is obviously an obsessional impulse: it is not unusual to find that such an individual has some compulsive action (these may be mental) as well to help control these urges. **[A. p309]**
84.4   **I.** Such panic attacks are frequently accompanied by fears that the individual is having a heart attack or brain haemorrhage, or is going mad. The individual will generally fear having another panic attack for some time afterwards as well. **[B. p86]**

85. Formal thought disorder
85.1   **B.** Here thoughts are associated by the sounds of words (rhyming) rather than their meaning. **[D. p658]**

85.2 **F.** Clang associations and flight of ideas are common in mania. **[D. p658]**

85.3 **J.** Here the patient gave a reply that is appropriate to the general topic without actually having answered the question. **[D. p658]**

85.4 **D.** There is a breakdown in both the logical connections between ideas and the overall sense of goal directedness. **[D. p658]**

86. Psychopathological features occasionally seen in schizophrenia

86.1 **E.** This knowledge of having a double is occasionally a delusion, or a hallucination as in this case (heautoscopy), but more commonly is a variant of a depersonalisation. **[A. p189–93]**

86.2 **B.** It is defined as at least a five-year difference between the patient's age and what he/she believes it to be. **[A. p66]**

86.3 **I.** This is rare now, but used to be seen more commonly in catatonic schizophrenia. **[A. p336]**

86.4 **D.** The written form of this is termed *cryptographia*. **[A. p159]**

87. Panic disorder

87.1 **C.** This is a common occurrence due to the patient's fear of loss of control. **[T. p476–7]**

87.2 **H.** Though the essential features of pure panic attacks are that they are non-situational and unexpected, a study reported that only 17% of panic attacks fulfilled this criteria. **[T. p476–7]**

87.3 **A.** They may last longer. **[T. p476–7]**

87.4 **J.** These secondary fears are almost always present. **[T. p476–7]**

88. First-rank symptoms of schizophrenia

88.1 **D.** The patient has had a real sensory experience in seeing the tractor, but this experience holds great meaning for him and his reading of the situation is clearly delusional. **[M. p124]**

88.2 **G.** The difficulty here is mainly in deciding what type of passivity phenomenon has taken place. While it may seem like a made action, the patient is stating that it is the *impulse* to do the action that has been implanted: if questioned, the patient will agree that the action in response to this was his own. **[A. p153]**

88.3 **J.** This is relatively straightforward, but one needs to be careful not to latch on to the word 'broadcasting' in the stem. Thoughts alien to the patient are being transmitted into his head and so this is thought insertion. **[M. p124]**

88.4 **H.** It is important to be able to differentiate somatic passivity from a haptic hallucination, since the latter is not a first-rank symptom. The sensation may be real or hallucinatory, but the patient explains it as being the result of the wishes of an external force. **[A. p153–4]**

89. Psychopathological terms from German psychiatry

89.1   **B.** Generally on the written papers these terms have their rough English translations beside them in brackets, but it is still important to try to know them in case they come up on their own or an examiner uses them in the vivas. It is easier to remember them if you take a little time to learn what the words mean in German. *Gedankenlautwerden* very roughly means: thoughts (*Gedanken*), loud (*laut*), to become (*werden*). **[A. p151]**

89.2   **D.** It is a motor disorder particularly associated with catatonic schizophrenia. The term means 'to go with' and it represents the extreme variant of *Mitmachen*. **[K. p89]**

89.3   **F.** The term means 'snout spasm' and can occur in neuroleptic-naïve patients. **[A. p337]**

89.4   **I.** *Wahn* means 'delusion' and *Stimmung* means 'mood'. *Delusional mood* has been used almost synonymously with the term *delusional atmosphere*. **[K. p84]**

90. Speech disorders

90.1   **J.** The patient clearly understands what the question means but gives an answer that is clearly incorrect. It is associated with hebephrenia and the Ganser syndrome. **[A. p60–1]**

90.2   **B.** These are sentences but they don't make any sense since there is a lack of logical connections. **[D. p658]**

90.3   **F.** Associated with Parkinson's disease, there is repetition of the last syllable of the last word. **[B. p85]**

91. Sensory distortions

91.1   **D.** This is not an unusual finding in delirium and it stresses the importance of addressing such patients in a loud, slow voice. **[A. p79]**

91.2   **B.** Macropsia and micropsia can also occur in epilepsy and other organic conditions. **[A. p79]**

91.3   **J.** Other sensory experiences can have lowered intensity in depression, such as a bland taste of food or loss of clarity for sounds. **[A. p79]**

91.4   **H.** This is a very uncommon occurrence, and is associated with schizophrenia and (more likely in this case) organic conditions. **[A. p80–1]**

92. Hallucinatory experiences

92.1   **J.** Autoscopy refers to seeing oneself as either a hallucinatory or pseudohallucinatory experience. Negative autoscopy is a variant of this in which the subject cannot see his reflection in a mirror. **[A. p95–6]**

92.2   **E.** Hallucinations of senations of the body have been divided into three categories: superficial, visceral and kinaesthetic. The first of these has been further subclassified into hygric, thermic and haptic. 'Hygric' refers to a fluid sensation in the body. **[A. p90]**

92.3   **L.** The main distinction between functional and reflex hallucinations is that the modalities of the stimulus and the hallucination are the same in the former and different in the latter. **[A. p96–7]**

92.4   **K.** This can refer also to duplication of parts of the body other than the limbs. **[K. p87]**

93. Disorders of mood and affect

93.1   **I.** The difficulty here is differentiating 'flattened' from 'blunted affect': the latter implies a degree of impairment of sensitivity to emotions. **[A. p277–8]**

93.2   **C.** Apathy often occurs along with anergia, and their meanings are sometimes confused. 'Apathy' is a word derived from the Greek: 'a' = without and 'pathos' = feeling. **[A. p277]**

93.3   **A.** This was described by Sifneos and is associated with conditions such as somatoform disorders, substance misuse and post-traumatic stress disorder. **[A. p281]**

93.4   **F.** Some factors may indicate an ecstatic experience to be more related to personal beliefs than psychopathology, such as a degree of reluctance to discuss the event and the understanding of the individual for others not being able to believe the experience. **[A. p283–4]**

94. Psychopathological features of delirium

94.1   **A.** It comes from a real perception, but is transformed, so it is an illusion. It can be seen as arising out of her emotional state, thus it is an affect illusion. When she settles and looks at the trolley she will see it for what it is; pareidolic illusions on the other hand become more defined with attention. **[A. p81–2]**

94.2   **C.** While these delusions are common, they tend not to be as elaborate as those seen in some of the functional psychotic disorders. **[C. p11]**

94.3   **B.** He is taking a literal, concrete meaning of the proverb. The speech of the delirious patient may also be speeded up, but even so, there is generally an impoverishment of content. **[C. p11]**

94.4   **L.** This is a form of disorientation of place. There is always some disorientation in delirium: that of time is most common. **[C. p11]**

95. Delusional disorder

95.1   **H.** Courbon and Tusques described this delusion in 1932. **[T. p440]**

95.2   **J.** Christodoulou described this in 1978. **[T. p440]**

95.3   **I.** This 'replacement' can be either physical, psychological or both. **[T. p440]**

95.4   **D.** Erotomania can present as a form of delusional disorder or as a symptom of schizophrenia or mania. **[T. p432–41]**

96. Psychodynamic theorists

96.1 **E, F, G.** Jung described complexes, but it is with Adler that the *inferiority complex* is most associated. According to him, individuals are born inferior and need to make efforts to combat this throughout life. This is associated with anxiety, particularly when efforts are thwarted. **[K. p75]**

96.2 **B, J, K.** Jung's theories are important but complex. Both the animus and the shadow are examples of his *archetypes*. *Synchronicity* forms part of his theory on causality. **[B. p99–100]**

96.3 **C, H.** Meyer wished to have a unified, clear approach to conceptualising and treating mental illness and stressed the importance of addressing the biopsychosocial model. **[K. p76]**

96.4 **I, L.** The *pathological mother* contrasts with the *good-enough mother* in that she puts her own needs before that of the child. The child thus has to create a *false self* as a defence. Other Winnicottian concepts include *transitional object, holding environment* and *potential space.* **[B. p102]**

97. Depersonalisation and derealisation

97.1 **F.** This has been described as an association of depersonalisation states. **[A. p206]**

97.2 **E.** The disturbance of awareness may involve individual organs. In the culture-bound syndrome *koro*, the fear of the penis shrinking and disappearing is an example of this. **[A. p206]**

97.3 **B.** The individual will experience his own mental processes to be strange. **[A. p206]**

97.4 **I.** The individual should know the object or situation, but feels strongly that he/she has never encountered it before. **[A. p206]**

98. Generalised anxiety disorder

98.1 **J.** Unlike obsessions, this thought is less intrusive and the content of the thought is acceptable. **[D. p1486–88]**

98.2 **B.** There is a blunted growth hormone response to clonidine challenge. **[D. p1453–88]**

98.3 **D.** Worrying, insecure attachment and conflict are thought to be important factors in the origin of the disorder. **[D. p1453–88]**

98.4 **G.** DSM-IV also requires the presence of symptoms for the same duration. **[D. p1453–88]**

99. Paranoid schizophrenia

99.1 **D.** First: since the voices are plotting together, they are referring him in the third person **[A. p149]**

99.2 **H.** Second-rank symptom, as these are not first-rank symptoms. **[A. p149]**

99.3 **C.** Freud suggested that the individual with paranoid thoughts denies his/her homosexual feelings and hatred and then projects the hatred to others. **[D. p602–3]**

99.4 **B.** The other psychopathologies associated with this stage are obsessions, compulsions, and impulsivity. **[D. p610]**

100. Pioneers of psychodynamic theory

100.1   **J.** The term 'character armour' should give this away. Reich's form of therapy was called *vegetotherapy* and is practised today as *bioenergetics*. **[D. p627–8]**

100.2   **A.** Adler rejected the notion of the libido theory as the root of all ills. He emphasised the importance of the influence of and interaction with society on the individual. Therapy involves inspecting one's lifestyle to see if there are discordances with social reality. **[D. p618–19]**

100.3   **F.** Sullivan is associated with the terms *prototaxic, parataxic* and *syntactic*. They denote differing modes of experiencing the environment. **[D. p633–5]**

101. Delusions

101.1   **E.** Both delusions are not understandable in the given context. **[A. p104]**

101.2   **C.** The ideas are vague and the uncertainty causes tension for the patient. She will be perplexed and apprehensive until the delusions become fully formed. **[A. p109–10]**

102. Auditory hallucinations

102.1   **F, H.** Generally, you will be told how many items you have to select for a given stem. This straightforward question is made slightly more difficult by leaving it to you to decide how many answers are needed. This phoneme is discussing what the patient does as she does it and refers to her in the third person. **[A. p151]**

102.2   **A, H.** Again, the patient is referred to in the third person, this time by two arguing voices. Running commentaries, arguing voices and audible thoughts are auditory hallucinations that are first-rank symptoms of schizophrenia. **[A. p151]**

102.3   **E.** The main distinction here is whether the thoughts spoken aloud occur as the patient thinks them, or whether there is a delay. Since they occur at the same time in this case, this is *Gedankenlautwerden* rather than *écho de pensée*. **[K. p86]**

102.4   **D.** Elementary hallucinations take the form of short grunts or whistles and are found in organic conditions such as delirium. **[K. p86]**

103. Delirium

103.1   **C.** Presence of autonomic disturbances, coarse tremors and visual and auditory hallucinations suggests this, rather than TLE. **[A. p30–1]**

103.2   **A.** These are complex coordinated actions taking place in impaired consciousness. **[A. p32–3]**

103.3   **H.** Lishman describes these characteristic features; duration can vary from a few hours to several weeks of the unexpected violence or emotional outbursts. **[A. p32]**

104. Disorders of consciousness

104.1   **D.** Drowsiness differs from clouding in degree: it is considered to be a higher step in the 'ladder' from alertness to coma. **[A. p28–9]**

104.2   **G.** This example of *occupational delirium* can be seen as an oneiroid state, as the patient here seems to be experiencing a 'dream-like' state. **[A. p33]**

104.3   **H.** There are three elements in the concept: abrupt onset, duration of hours to weeks and violence or marked emotional reactions occurring out of the blue. **[A. p32]**

104.4   **F.** The amount of alcohol involved can vary and sometimes only very modest amounts are involved. **[A. p34–5]**

105. Perceptual disorder

105.1   **F, I.** The phenomenology of auditory hallucinations has much importance for diagnosis. Voices that speak the patient's thoughts aloud, give a running commentary, or speak to each other, are most commonly associated with schizophrenia. **[A. p85]**

105.2   **G.** Organic auditory hallucinations, when they take the form of voices, are usually short utterances in the second person. **[A. p85]**

105.3   **E.** In linguistics, phonemes are the units of speech sound, which is a completely different meaning. Morphemes are the meaningful parts of words. The term 'hallucineme' is nonsense. **[A. p86]**

106. Alcoholism and cognitive impairment

106.1   **G.** Korsakoff's psychosis is associated with two forms of confabulation. Best-known is the fantastic confabulation, in which the patient describes fantastic adventures with little prompting. Suggestibility is a prominent feature of Korsakoff's. **[A. p52–3]**

106.2   **B.** On the other hand, in confabulation of embarrassment, the patient reveals social awareness and some realisation of social requirements. **[A. p53]**

106.3   **L.** This tends to be a striking finding in the confabulating patient **[A. p53–4]**

106.4   **H.** Korsakoff's psychosis is associated with medial diencephalon injury (which includes the mammiliary bodies) and patients often have frontal lobe damage as well. **[D. p430]**

107. Methods of controlling thoughts and impulses

107.1   **A.** Temporarily inhibiting thinking closely resembles repression, but in *blocking* distress arises when the thought is inhibited. **[D. p584]**

107.2   **J.** The issue is not avoided but it is consciously postponed. **[D. p585]**

107.3 **H.** Withholding ideas, once consciously experienced, is termed *secondary repression*, whereas the curbing of ideas before one is consciously aware of them is termed *primary repression*. **[D. p582–5]**

107.4 **E.** The thoughts are isolated and repressed from the associated affect and hence she continues to experience anxiety but she is unaware of the disturbing thoughts. **[D. p582–5]**

108. Object relations

108.1 **I.** Mothers should be 'good enough' to allow the child's healthy protest about parental failure: in this way the infant learns to develop his own strengths to cope with such situations. **[E. p350–1]**

108.2 **E.** The 'ideal object' is one that would never cause frustration, while the 'antilibidinal object' is one that causes frustration. **[E. p350]**

108.3 **B.** The paranoid-schizoid position involves splitting, blaming and avoidance. **[E. p348–50]**

108.4 **G.** Here the initially injured party communicates pain indirectly by inducing those feelings in the other by means of projective identification. **[E. p349]**

109. Psychodynamics of depression

109.1 **C.** He felt that such self-criticism and lowered self-esteem in depressed patients are not directed at the self but rather at an introject of some object. **[D. p599]**

109.2 **G.** At the same time, they long for the lost love object. **[D. p599]**

Clinical Theory and Skills EMIs

110. Conducting the psychiatric interview

110.1   **B.** Despite this and other psychiatric jargon having entered common usage, it is important to explore exactly what the patient means by the term: it frequently varies considerably from what you understand by it. **[D. p660–5]**

110.2   **J.** It is important to find out how the patient wishes to be addressed: if in doubt, few will take offence at using their title, and they will generally tell you to use their first name if this is what they want. It looks poor in the clinical examination if the patient/actor corrects you in front of the examiners because you have not taken this into consideration. **[D. p660–5]**

110.3   **E.** It looks callous if you do not, although the reaction need not be direct or even verbal: an appropriate sympathetic look while offering a tissue might suffice, although something like 'you seem very upset...' may help the patient express why she is distressed. The artificiality of feigned empathy is generally spotted and does little to build rapport. **[D. p660–5]**

110.4   **A.** It is good practice to get into the habit of asking for a chaperone regularly whether you are male or female: not all situations in which you will need one will be signposted in advance. **[D. p660–5]**

111. ICD–10 diagnoses

111.1   **I.** Though he developed these symptoms following bereavement, the depressive symptoms are severe and new symptoms have developed recently. **[X. p123–4]**

111.2   **B.** This is a diagnosable disorder in ICD-10 (F38.10). **[X. p131]**

111.3   **D.** Dysthymia can persist indefinitely and, along with cyclothymia, is one of the two named persistent mood disorders in ICD-10. **[X. p129–30]**

112. Concepts of schizophrenia

112.1   **B.** This is one of Bleuler's four As: Autism, Ambivalence, Affective incongruity, and loosening of Associations. **[M. p120]**

112.2   **E.** Hearing her thoughts spoken aloud is thought echo. **[M. p124]**

112.3   **D.** Krapelin based his theories on organic factors. **[D. p1096]**

112.4   **G.** Bleuler was influenced by Freud to arrive at this hypothesis. **[D. p1096]**

113. Clinical progression of dementias

113.1 **A.** The triad consisting of progressive dementia, pyramidal and extrapyramidal symptoms, myoclonus and the characteristic triphasic waves is highly suggestive of this disease. **[X. p52–3]**

113.2 **C.** Huntington's disease is transmitted by a single autosomal dominant gene. The association of choreiform movements, dementia and a positive family history is highly suggestive of this diagnosis. **[X. p53–4]**

113.3 **F.** The presence of hypertension, good insight, and unevenly impaired cognitive functions suggests vascular dementia. CT brain studies may be useful in confirming the diagnosis. **[X. p50–1]**

114. Interviewing the patient

114.1 **B.** They are best evaluated with a respectful but somewhat distant formality, and with scrupulous honesty. **[D. p662]**

114.2 **A.** Although depressed patients should not be badgered, long silences are seldom useful. Ruminative patients will need to be interrupted and redirected. **[D. p662–3]**

114.3 **E.** The interviewer must attempt not to be provocative and to avoid promising outcomes in exchange for cooperation. **[D. p663]**

114.4 **F.** Patient need not try to seduce the doctor physically: money or information may be offered. It is important to firmly refuse such offers in a sympathetic way so that patients do not feel ashamed afterwards, else the therapeutic relationship will be affected. **[D. p664]**

115. Schizophrenia

115.1 **B.** Hebephrenic schizophrenia usually starts between the ages of 15 and 25 and tends to have a poor prognosis. **[X. p90–1]**

115.2 **C.** As there is yet a prominent, florid schizophrenia picture, the diagnosis of post-schizophrenic depression is not made. Since the duration of depressive symptoms is only a week and there are only a few depressive symptoms, this also rules out post-schizophrenic depression and schizoaffective disorder. **[X. p93–4]**

115.3 **A.** The prominent features are excitement and posturing; the presence of other catatonic features will confirm the diagnosis. **[X. p91–2]**

116. Dementia

116.1 **C.** Hirano bodies and Lewy bodies may also be found. However, Lewy bodies are not specific to Alzheimer's disease and may be associated with conditions such as Parkinson's disease. **[T. p292–3]**

116.2 **E.** In Parkinson's disease, cortical Lewy bodies are at lower densities than in dementia of the Lewy body type, while there is much more extensive nigral dopaminergic neuronal loss (80% versus 40–60% respectively). **[T. p300–1]**

116.3   **F.** One hypothesis for the abnormal movements seen in Huntington's disease is the imbalance between the functioning of GABA (γ-aminobutyric acid) and dopamine. **[T. p290–300]**

117. Anxiety disorders in DSM–IV

117.1   **F.** This is one differentiating feature of DSM-IV from ICD-10. In DSM-IV, panic disorder is considered higher on the hierarchy, so that if one has ever had a history of panic disorder, one cannot be diagnosed as having agoraphobia alone. Panic disorder is sub-classified as being with or without agoraphobia. **[O. p402–3]**

117.2   **I.** This is the *blood–injection–injury* subtype of specific phobia. It contrasts with the other subtypes in that the patient's blood pressure tends to drop and patients can often faint. It also tends to have a strong family history. **[O. p406–7]**

117.3   **C.** While this is suggestive of OCD, the symptoms neither cause 'marked distress', take up a significant amount of time (more than an hour) or appear to interfere greatly with her psychosocial functioning. **[O. p423]**

117.4   **H.** A tricky one, this: while this might seem to be a specific phobia, DSM-IV recognises that culture can have a pathoplastic effect on clinical presentation. People from areas such as Japan and Korea may have concerns about giving offence to others rather than social embarrassment in social phobia. **[O. p413]**

118. Anorexia nervosa

118.1   **I.** Individuals with anorexia nervosa rarely starve to be attractive to others. **[T. p513]**

118.2   **D.** They tend to gauge the size of other people and inanimate objects correctly but not their own size. **[T. p514]**

118.3   **F.** Vitamin deficiencies are uncommon. **[T. p517]**

118.4   **A.** This is responsible for the feelings of fullness. **[T. p517]**

119. Social causation of schizophrenia

119.1   **G.** Lidz described marital schism and skew. Schism refers to overt conflict in the marriage with consequent difficulties for the child being put into the position of taking sides. **[B. p74]**

119.2   **C.** Bates felt that such impossible situations caused the child to retreat and later, possibly, develop schizophrenia. As with other such theories, it perpetuated the idea for some in the public that families are 'to blame' for schizophrenia. **[K. p63]**

119.3   **J.** While this does have overlap with expressed emotion, indifference has not generally been described with the latter. Fromm-Reichman described the *schizophrenogenic mother* and attributed such traits, as well as distance and rejecting attitudes, to her. **[K. p63]**

119.4   **B.** The breeder hypothesis contrasts with the drifter hypothesis in that the latter postulates that differences in incidence of schizophrenia across socio-economic groups and areas relate to a downward social drift of those suffering as their performance is impaired by the illness. **[M. p123]**

120. *Clinical manifestations of somatoform disorders*

120.1 **H.** In somatisation disorder there is usually excessive medication use, together with non-compliance over long periods. **[X. p162–4]**

120.2 **E.** Hypochondriacal patients seek reassurance by frequent visits to different physicians. **[X. p164–6]**

120.3 **I.** In generalised anxiety disorder, on the other hand, there will be a preoccupation with the psychological accompaniments of autonomic arousal such as fear. **[X. p166–8]**

121. *Paraphilias*

121.1 **K.** This fantasy of shaming the observed victim is common in voyeurism. **[A. p250]**

121.2 **C.** Such individuals generally fantasize that they are having an intimate, mutual sexual relationship with the individual they are rubbing up against. **[E. p902]**

121.3 **F.** While this is a variant of fetishism, it is more properly termed *partialism*, since individuals are excited by a part of the body, rather than by an inanimate object. **[E. p902]**

121.4 **A.** The differential here from the options list is *public masturbation*. The latter however involves the individual hiding his penis while he watches a woman and masturbates. **[E. p904]**

122. *Physical signs*

122.1 **F.** This is a roughened area of skin generally over the back of metacarpal-phalangeal joints of the 2nd or 3rd digits, or more proximal, and comes from this area rubbing the teeth when the digits are used to induce vomiting. **[N. p886]**

122.2 **E.** This is a characteristic folding of the brow associated with depressive syndromes: its name comes from the fold's resemblance to the Greek alphabet character omega (Ω). **[D. p1504]**

122.3 **D.** This sign suggests meningism, but is not always present. It involves passive extension of the knee when the hip is flexed. **[C. p365]**

122.4 **B, H.** The most likely diagnosis is an insidious onset hypopara-thyroidism. The hypocalcaemia may be revealed by tapping the facial nerve slightly before the tragus, which pulls the mouth towards your finger (Chvostek's sign), or by revealing *main d'accoucheur* by inflating a sphygmomanometer cuff above systolic pressure on the arm (Trousseau's sign). **[C. p531–3]**

123. Disorders in old age

123.1   **G.** The terminology of this condition is confusing at times. The quoted text draws a distinction between 'late-onset' (40–60 years) schizophrenia, which more resembles early onset, and 'very-late-onset' (onset after 60), while other authors use *late-onset schizophrenia* or *paraphrenia* to denote the latter. The main differential in the above is delusional disorder, but the presence of the *partition delusion* (believing that organisms or substances can pass through impenetrable barriers) suggests late-onset schizophrenia. Negative symptoms are rare in this condition. **[E. p1641–4]**

123.2   **E.** Elderly and younger patients tend to have broadly similar symptoms of depression. The elderly tend to have more hypochondriacal concerns, agitation and depressive delusions. Despite this, it is still imperative that this patient be investigated thoroughly to exclude a physical disorder, as depression commonly coexists with physical illness in this population. **[E. p1644–5]**

123.3   **H.** In the past it was suggested that the elderly tend to get more mixed patterns than classical manic symptoms. It has been found, however, that although mania is rare in this group, patients can get the same range of symptoms as do the young. Remember that elated mood may not be present in mania: some patients mainly display irritability. **[E. p1650]**

124. Organic disorders

124.1   **J.** Excess T_4 and/or T_3 will establish if hyperthyroidism is present. **[T. p321–2]**

124.2   **F.** The psychiatric disturbances are usually resolved with treatment of the underlying disorder. **[T. p322]**

124.3   **A.** Addison's disease results from deficient production of corticosteroids by the adrenal gland. **[T. p322–3]**

125. Patterns of behaviour in personality disorders

125.1   **B.** The other cluster C personality disorders are dependent personality disorder and obsessive-compulsive personality disorder. **[O. p662–5]**

125.2   **C.** The other cluster B personality disorders are antisocial personality disorder, histrionic personality disorder and narcissistic personality disorder. **[O. p650–4]**

125.3   **G.** The other cluster A personality disorders are schizoid personality disorder and schizotypal personality disorder. **[O. p634–8]**

126. Sleep disturbances in psychiatric disorders

126.1   **E.** In panic disorder, nocturnal panic attacks occur during non-REM sleep. **[E. p1021–5]**

126.2   **B.** The most widely reported finding has been the reduced latency to REM sleep onset. Patients with manic or eating disorders show similar sleep abnormalities, but the evidence is not as strong as for depression. Patients with dysthymia are indistinguishable from normal controls. **[E. p1021–5]**

126.3   **D.** Chronic alcohol use tends to produce loss of slow wave sleep. **[E. p1021–5]**

126.4   **A.** As stimulants suppress REM sleep the withdrawal is characterised by REM sleep rebound. **[E. p1021–5]**

127. Delirium

127.1   **I.** Nocturnal agitation is very common. **[T. p287]**

127.2   **H.** Such patients are particularly prone to anticholinergic effects, which must be borne in mind when prescribing drugs such as procyclidine or tricyclic antidepressants. **[T. p288–9]**

127.3   **C.** But commonly in delirium, many neurotransmitters are affected. **[T. p289]**

127.4   **F.** Long-term memory is disturbed in very severe cases. **[T. p287]**

128. Hierarchical structure of diagnosis in ICD–10

128.1   **F.** There is empirical justification for this arrangement as the patient's prognosis depends on the most severe diagnosis. **[T. p272]**

128.2   **D.** Hence a diagnosis of schizophrenia cannot be made if the patient also fulfils affective disorder criteria, unless the symptoms of schizophrenia predated the affective symptoms. **[T. p271]**

128.3   **B.** At the top of the hierarchy are the organic syndromes. **[T. p271]**

128.4   **I.** Foulds suggested that this similarity is because of the nature of symptoms of psychiatric illness. **[T. p272]**

129. DSM–IV personality disorder criteria

129.1   **C, D.** While many with antisocial personality lack empathy for others, this trait is listed specifically only for narcissistic personality disorder. **[O. p649–50]**

129.2   **F, H.** Both of these traits, in moderation, can confer advantages in certain situations, as indeed can many of the traits listed in the diagnostic criteria for the personality disorders. It is important to remember the general criterion for diagnosing personality disorders, that the '…pattern leads to clinically significant distress or impairment'. **[O. p633, 772–3]**

129.3   **G, J.** One differentiating feature of schizoid and paranoid personality disordered patients is that the former tend to be unaffected by either praise or criticism, while the latter react very negatively when criticised. **[O. p637–8]**

129.4   **A, D.** Impulsivity is a trait shared with antisocial personality, and highlights the reality that personality disordered patients often satisfy criteria for more than one of such discrete categories. **[O. p654]**

130. Sleep disorders and parasomnias

130.1   **G.** He has a number of the components of narcolepsy, which include: narcoleptic attacks, excessive daytime tiredness, cataplexy, hypnagogic hallucinations (less commonly hypnopompic) and sleep paralysis. **[A. p43]**

130.2   **F.** This is a rare condition. High voltage δ waves on the EEG are seen and the subject can be woken normally from the sleeping periods. **[M. p140]**

130.3   **J.** As a result of the obesity, this patient has apnoeic periods at night, resulting in the marked tiredness during the day. **[A. p42]**

130.4   **I.** One of the distinguishing factors between night terrors and nightmares is that the events of the former are not remembered as they occur in non-REM sleep. Enuresis is occasionally found to be associated with night terrors. **[B. p333–4]**

131. Alcohol use disorders

131.1   **E.** The female body has a lower ratio of water to fat. **[T. p340]**

131.2   **G.** In other words, one-in-three of the patients with alcohol dependence you will see are women. **[T. p340]**

131.3   **C.** There is an excess of male heavy drinkers either in her biological family or among the partners in her relationship history. **[T. p340]**

131.4   **J.** Although it is not known if it is more common in patients with alcohol dependence than in patients with other conditions. **[T. p340]**

132. Culture–bound syndromes

132.1   **C.** While this behaviour obviously could describe *amok*, the term used in Polynesia is *cathard* (or *cafard*). *Amok* is particularly described among inhabitants of Malaysia, while a similar syndrome is termed *Iich'aa* among the Navaho. **[D. p466–7]**

132.2   **E.** *Koro* is more commonly known to refer to the sudden fear in a male that his penis is retracting up into his abdomen (sometimes up into the brain) and that this will kill him. A female form is recognised where the retracting organs are the nipples or the vulva. **[D. p1272]**

132.3   **K.** Associated with severe depressive states, the delusion in *windigo* causes the individual to think that he/she has turned into a beast with cannibalistic tendencies. **[S. p387]**

132.4   **J.** *Susto* is associated with conditions such as post-traumatic stress disorder, depression or somatoform disorder. The individual may have a number of anxiety or depressive symptoms as well as a variety of physical symptoms. *Zar*, on the other hand, refers to the belief of being possessed by a spirit held by some individuals from North-West Africa or the Middle East. **[D. p1273]**

133. Depression in the postpartum period
133.1   **C.** ICD-10 discourages one from categorising such disorders as postnatal depression as a separate entity. **[T. p557–9]**
133.2   **H.** As this episode is not part of a non-postpartum recurrent depressive disorder. **[T. p557–9]**
133.3   **B.** The risk of developing further depression in the postpartum period was found to be 41% in one study among women who had no previous history of depression. **[T. p557–9]**
133.4   **F.** In these societies socio-cultural rituals clearly define the expected behaviour of the new mother as well as providing structured social support. **[T. p557–9]**

134. Psychotherapy
134.1   **G.** IPT is not as theory-driven as many other psychotherapies. It notes that depression is related to interpersonal difficulties and aims to help the individual address these to relieve symptoms. The initial stage involves framing the problems in one of four areas: role dispute, role transition, grief or interpersonal deficits. **[D. p2178–80]**
134.2   **B.** Brief individual psychodynamic psychotherapy differs from psychoanalytic psychotherapy in that sessions total only 10–20 on average, as its name suggests. Because of this, large-scale attempts at personal restructuring are not attempted. Instead, manageable, focused goals are identified and adhered to throughout the sessions, otherwise there is a danger that it will transmute into a long-term therapy. Brief psychodynamic psychotherapy is more likely than cognitive-analytic therapy to be the answer in this case as there is little mention in the stem of attention to concepts of cognitive theory. **[E. p1427–9]**
134.3   **E.** Various techniques from the psychotherapies may of course be used in the counselling to help achieve such goals. Thus variations on the central themes of counselling include interpersonal counselling, psychodynamic counselling and problem-solving counselling. **[E. p1361–2]**

135. Psychoanalysis
135.1   **E.** Such motor symptoms are generally worse when the patient is observed. **[D. 1510t]**
135.2   **F.** Free association is the typical therapeutic technique used to analyse the patient. **[D. p563–71]**
135.3   **A.** This is the main mechanism that brings resolution of symptoms. **[D. p563–71]**

135.4   **J.** Transference refers to the patient acting, feeling or behaving towards the therapist in ways that reflect ways of interacting with a significant other from the past. **[D. p563–71]**

136. Mood disorders in DSM–IV
136.1   **D.** The College indicates that candidates need only have a detailed knowledge of either ICD-10 or DSM-IV and a familiarity with the other. Despite the widespread use of ICD-10 in Ireland and Britain, it is common to get MCQs requiring detailed knowledge of DSM-IV. It is prudent therefore to have a good knowledge of DSM-IV for the written exams at the very least. Note that with cyclothymic disorder, after the initial two years' history required, if another mood disorder appears, such as a manic episode, then the appropriate diagnosis can be given as well (e.g. bipolar I disorder) comorbid with the cyclothymic disorder. **[O. p365]**
136.2   **J.** To give a diagnosis of a mixed episode in DSM-IV, criteria for both mania and major depression must be fulfilled for at least a week. **[O. p335]**
136.3   **L.** Since this episode of hypomania is likely to have resulted from a somatic treatment of depression, it does not count towards a diagnosis of bipolar II disorder. The current mood disorder would best be termed a substance-induced mood disorder. **[O. p359]**

137. ICD–10 classification of anxiety disorders
137.1   **G.** *Social neurosis* is the other term included under social phobias. **[X. p137–9]**
137.2   **A.** If social phobia is severe, there are often elements of depression and agoraphobia. **[X. p137–8]**
137.3   **C.** F40.00 is agoraphobia without panic disorder, while F40.01 is agoraphobia with panic disorder. This higher placing of agoraphobia in the hierarchy contrasts with DSM-IV. **[X. p134–9]**
137.4   **H.** This also includes acrophobia, animal phobias and examination phobia. **[X. p134–9]**

138. Diagnosing personality disorders using DSM–IV
138.1   **A, C, F, G.** A number of questions on personality disorders have been presented in this book, as this is a likely subject for examination by EMI: these questions need to have a list of options, and personality disorders eminently suit this requirement. The listed conditions here are the four that make up the DSM-IV Cluster B personality disorders. **[O. p645]**

138.2   **I, K, L.** Despite his general practitioner's views, it appears that the patient may have one or more conditions from the DSM-IV Cluster A personality disorders; these have been enduring since his teenage years. Having few contacts and a constricted affect suggest schizoid or schizotypal disorders, His suspiciousness also suggests schizotypal disorder and, of course, paranoid personality disorder. The latter is also suggested by his reluctance to confide (and possibly by the opened letter from his general practitioner). **[O. p637–8, 641, 645]**

138.3   **L.** There are a number of features in this additional information that are suggestive of schizotypal personality disorder: magical thinking, vague speech, peculiar appearance and probable excessive social anxiety. A psychotic disorder would need to be ruled out, but it appears that these difficulties are longstanding and part of the patient's personality structure. Schizotypal personality disorder has a prevalence of about 3% in the general population and patients, as in borderline personality disorder, can have brief psychotic episodes, especially during times of stress. **[O. p641–5]**

139. Complications of excessive alcohol

139.1   **H.** Wernickes's encephalopathy has ocular palsy. Polyneuropathy does not involve the cranial nerves. **[T. p346–7]**

139.2   **E.** Steatosis is fat deposition in liver cells: normal LFTs do not preclude its presence. **[T. p347]**

139.3   **G.** This is thought to be due to accelerated gastric emptying. **[T. p347]**

139.4   **I.** Such arrhythmias are sometimes known as the *holiday heart syndrome.* **[T. p347]**

140. Dementia syndromes

140.1   **B.** This is also known as subcortical arteriosclerotic encephalopathy. Key diagnostic features are: the history of hypertension, the neurological deficits (such as the pseudobulbar palsy) and subcortical, but little cortical, abnormalities on radiology. **[C. p458–9]**

140.2   **J.** The latter are the Pick bodies and these are evident on autopsy, along with 'knife-blade' atrophy of the gyri of the frontal and temporal regions. It can be difficult to differentiate Pick's disease from frontotemporal dementia clinically, and it is in fact uncertain how distinct they are as conditions. **[C. p460–3]**

140.3   **H.** This is an uncommon but important cause of dementia as it may be treatable. It should be suspected with the coinciding of the progressive subcortical dementia along with gait changes or urinary incontinence. Removing about 30 ml of cerebrospinal fluid may lead to improvement of symptoms for a while. **[C. p744–7]**

141. Bipolar affective disorder

141.1   **A.** These disturbances are due to changes of affect. **[D. p398–9]**

141.2   **G.** Valproate increases the levels of lamotrigine and thus increases the risk of developing a pruritic rash. **[D. p1404]**

141.3   **J.** As his depression is mild an SSRI should be avoided, as aggressive treatment with an antidepressant could destabilise the course of illness. **[D. p732]**

141.4   **B.** In bipolar II disorder, the manic symptoms are mild and do not manifest in more severe forms than a hypomanic episode. It is important to remember that the presence of psychotic symptoms in an elation means that the episode is a manic one, whatever the severity of the other symptoms (assuming organic causes have been outruled). **[D. p1359–63]**

142. Psychopathology of endocrine disorders

142.1   **A.** The usual cause is a tumour of the anterior pituitary. Psychotic symptoms can occur but are generally rare. **[N. p1151]**

142.2   **C.** The depression can be marked in some patients. Depressive symptoms are the most common psychiatric manifestation and are more common with pituitary causes than adrenal causes of Cushing's syndrome. **[N. p1146–7]**

142.3   **E.** Other psychiatric manifestations of hyperthyroidism are generally uncommon and include psychosis and delirium. **[N. p1141–4]**

143. Correlates of outcome in schizophrenia

143.1   **A, D, E, F.** This is another list of factors that you need to know well for both the MCQs and OSCE. Other good prognostic indicators include female sex, higher socio-economic status and not having negative symptoms. **[M. p131]**

143.2   **C, H, I, J.** These are mostly the converse of the factors associated with good prognosis, and include: long duration of untreated psychosis (DUP), cognitive impairment and living in developed countries. **[M. p131]**

143.3   **B, G, H.** Non-concordance is a serious problem in schizophrenia since it is one of the very few prognostic factors that can be addressed. Poor insight, side-effects and poor efficacy are among the factors that may limit concordance. **[B. p260]**

143.4   **A, C, F, I.** Depressive symptoms, male sex and unemployment are associated with risk of suicide in general, and have been confirmed as risk factors for suicide in schizophrenia. Side-effects of medication might be expected to be associated with an increased risk, but it is akathisia that has been most implicated. Those with paranoid schizophrenia are at three times the risk of those with other subtypes. **[B. p261–2, M. p131–2]**

144. Sequelae of alcohol abuse

144.1   **G.** This is obviously a rare condition. While some patients may recover, others may progress to coma and die. **[E. p491]**

144.2 **H.** Since only a proportion of individuals with thiamine deficiency go on to develop Wernicke's, it is hypothesised that such individuals may have deficiencies in the biochemical pathways for thiamine utilisation. **[E. p491]**

144.3 **B.** The main difficulty in this item is recognising that 'alcohol-induced psychosis' is another term for 'delirium tremens'. **[E. p489]**

144.4 **D.** Apart from the quadriplegia and bulbar palsy, patients can develop loss of pain sensation. The demyelination is in the pons, as the name suggests, and the condition is frequently fatal. Too fast a correction of hyponatraemia has been suggested as one cause, as has dietary deficiencies. **[C. p586]**

145. Movement disorders

145.1 **G.** In adults, hemiathetosis is associated with lesions of the putamen. **[Q. p78]**

145.2 **I.** Ballism is associated with lesions of the subthalamic nucleus. **[Q. p78]**

145.3 **E.** Tics are associated with dopamine abnormalities but no consistent pathologic abnormality has been demonstrated for these disorders. **[Q. p78]**

145.4 **H.** Adult-form chorea is associated with striatal degeneration. **[Q. p78]**

146. Psychotic and related disorders in ICD-10

146.1 **G.** Since marked affective symptoms developed soon *after* the onset of the psychotic symptoms and remain significant throughout the illness alongside the psychotic symptoms. The psychotic symptoms themselves alone fulfil criteria for a diagnosis of schizophrenia. The affective symptoms are consistent with a manic pattern. **[X. p105–7]**

146.2 **C.** The most striking symptom is the persistent delusion. Other areas of his life appear largely intact, and there are no symptoms particularly suggestive of schizophrenia. Brief depressive symptoms do not invalidate the diagnosis. His depressive symptoms appear to be of relatively recent onset in the course of his illness. **[X. p97–9]**

146.3 **I.** The most likely diagnosis is schizotypal disorder. Clearly there are a number of features of this disorder: circumstantial speech, aloofness, odd appearance and a transient psychotic-like period. It appears from collateral history that such disturbances are long-standing. **[X. p95–6]**

147. Neuropsychiatric sequelae of multiple sclerosis

147.1 **F.** In the course of multiple sclerosis, half of patients will develop a major depressive episode. **[T. p320]**

147.2 **D.** Euphoria occurs in 10% of patients: severe cognitive impairment is usually found when this occurs. **[T. p320]**

147.3   **B.** Another fact that supports the notion of a genetic vulnerability for MS is that the monozygotic to dizygotic twin concordance is 30% versus 4%. **[T. p320]**

147.4   **J.** Dementia commonly occurs late in the course of the illness and occasionally has a rapid progression. **[T. p320]**

148. Sequelae of vitamin deficiencies

148.1   **K.** He is suffering from pellagra, caused mainly by a lack of nicotinic acid in his diet. Obviously rare in affluent societies, there is a classic triad of symptoms described: skin lesions, gastrointestinal disturbance and psychiatric symptoms. The latter can include delirium, memory impairment and psychotic symptoms. **[C. p571–3; D. p2523]**

148.2   **B.** It must be borne in mind that Wernicke's encephalopathy may be caused by conditions other than alcoholism: in this case hyperemesis gravidarum. The classic triad of confusion, ataxia and ophthalmoplegia are present in this scenario. **[C. p575–82]**

148.3   **E.** Similar psychiatric symptomatology may be caused by vitamin B_{12} and folate deficiencies. In this scenario a deficiency of the former is more likely since the physical signs and laboratory results are consistent with pernicious anaemia, the most common cause of reduced B_{12} levels in the elderly. **[C. p587–90; D. p735–44,1811]**

148.4   **J.** Anticonvulsant therapy, especially that with phenytoin, is associated with reduced serum and red-cell folate levels. Folate deficiency has been associated with depressive symptoms, dementia and occasionally psychotic symptoms. Poor dietary intake associated with alcohol abuse is a more common cause of reduced folate levels. **[C. p590–3; D. p2523]**

149. The electroencephalogram (EEG)

149.1   **L.** These complexes have a frequency of about 1 Hz and occur in virtually all such patients. **[K. p141]**

149.2   **H, I.** A diffuse flattening of the EEG tracing is also seen. δ and θ activity are unusual in the normal, awake adult. **[K. p141]**

149.3   **A, G, I.** This is a class effect of benzodiazepines. Barbiturates also cause this but can also give rise to the occasional δ wave. **[M. p139]**

149.4   **None.** At therapeutic levels lithium causes very few EEG changes but increased δ/θ activity can be seen with toxicity. Don't worry overly about this answer, however: there won't be any trick questions in the real exam. **[B. p145]**

150. Phenotypic similarities between Axis I and Axis II disorders

150.1   **E.** The distinction is whether such symptoms are *states* (Axis I) or *traits* (Axis II) in the individual. **[D. p1750–1]**

150.2   **A.** Many authors believe that these are alternative labels for the same conditions. **[D. p1750–1]**

150.3 **E.** Narcissistic, histrionic and antisocial personality disorders are considered as minor variants of cyclothymia, bipolar disorder and mania, based on these features. **[D. p1750–1]**

150.4 **B.** Hypochondriasis and inflexibility are shared symptoms of OCD and obsessive-compulsive personality disorder. **[D. p1750–1]**

References

Note: References in the answer section are given in the format: **[G. p136]**. This indicates that the topic relating to that particular answer may be found on page 136 of the text listed at 'G' below.

A.   Sims A. *Symptoms in the Mind: An Introduction to Descriptive Psychopathology,* 2nd edn. London: WB Saunders Company Ltd, 1995.

B.   Puri BK, Hall AD. *Revision Notes in Psychiatry.* London: Arnold, 1998.

C.   Lishman WA. *Organic Psychiatry,* 3rd edn. Oxford: Blackwell Science, 1998.

D.   Sadock BJ, Sadock VA (editors). *Kaplan & Sadock's Comprehensive Textbook of Psychiatry,* 7th edn. Philadelphia (PA): Lippincott Williams & Wilkins, 2000.

E.   Gelder MG, López-Ibor JJ, Andreasen N (editors). *New Oxford Textbook of Psychiatry.* Oxford: Oxford University Press, 2000.

F.   British Medical Association and the Royal Pharmaceutical Society of Great Britain. *British National Formulary.* Number 42. London: The Pharmaceutical Press, 2001.

G.   Cookson J, Taylor D, Katona C. *Use of Drugs in Psychiatry,* 5th edn. London: Gaskell, 2002.

H.   Taylor D, Paton C, Kerwin R. *The South London & Maudsley NHS Trust 2003 Prescribing Guidelines,* 7th edn. London: Martin Dunitz, 2003.

I.   Bazire S. *Psychotropic Drug Directory 2001/02: the Professionals' Pocket Handbook & Aide Memoire.* Salisbury: Quay Books, 2001.

J.   Gross R. *Psychology: The Science of Mind and Behaviour,* 4th edn. London: Hodder & Stoughton, 2001.

K.   Malhi GS, Mitchell AJ. *Examination Notes in Psychiatry, Basic Sciences: A Postgraduate Text.* Oxford: Butterworth-Heinemann, 1999.

L.   Eysenck M. *Simply Psychology.* Hove: Psychology Press, 1996.

M.   Lawlor BA (editor). *Revision Psychiatry.* Dublin: MedMedia Ltd, 2001.

N.   Stein G, Wilkinson G (editors). *Seminars in General Adult Psychiatry.* London: Gaskell, 1998.

O.   American Psychiatric Association. *Diagnostic and Statistical Manual of Mental Disorders, Fourth Edition: DSM-IV.* Washington (DC): American Psychiatric Association, 1994.

P.   Stahl SM. *Essential Psychopharmacology: Neuroscientific Basis and Practical Applications,* 2nd edn. Cambridge: Cambridge University Press, 2000.

Q.   Carpenter R. *Neurophysiology,* 4th edn. London: Hodder Arnold, 2002.

R.   Liebert RM, Liebert LL. *Liebert & Spiegler's Personality Strategies and Issues,* 8th edn. Pacific Grove (CA): Brooks/Cole, 1998.

S.   Buckley P, Bird J, Harrison G. *Examination Notes in Psychiatry: a Postgraduate Text,* 3rd edn. Oxford: Butterworth-Heinemann, 1995.

T.   Johnstone EC, Freeman CPL, Zealley AK (editors). *Companion to Psychiatric Studies,* 6th edn. London: Churchill Livingstone, 1998.

U.   Brown D, Pedder J. *Introduction to Psychotherapy: an Outline of Psychodynamic Principles and Practice,* 2nd edn. London: Routledge, 1991.

V.   King DJ. *Seminars in Clinical Psychopharmacology.* London: Gaskell, 1995.

W.   Stahl SM. *Psychopharmacology of Antidepressants.* London: Martin Dunitz, 1999.

X.   World Health Organisation. *The ICD-10 Classification of Mental and Behavioural Disorders: Clinical Descriptions and Diagnostic Guidelines.* Geneva: World Health Organisation, 1992.

Y.   Coon D. *Essentials of Psychology: Exploration and Application,* 7th edn. London: Brooks/Cole, 1997.

Index of Questions

Note: The numbers refer to the question number, not the page number.

aggression 4, 9
agnosias 12
alcohol abuse 131
  sequelae 139, 144
  cognitive impairment 106
anorexia nervosa 118
anticholinergics 64
antidepressants 55
  adverse effects 53, 59, 63
  MAOIs 70
  newer antidepressants 50, 72
  receptor changes 46, 57, 66
antipsychotics
  adverse effects 40, 41, 43, 48, 73
  atypical 45, 68
  emergencies 39
anxiety disorders
  DSM-IV 117
  ICD-10 137
  psychopathology 84
anxiolytics
  hypnotics 47, 62
  pharmacodynamics 58, 60
attachment 22
attraction 15

behaviour
  analysis 35
  modification 21
  theory 32
  therapy 33
  prosocial 28
bipolar affective disorder 141
  perceptual abnormalities 83

clozapine 52
culture-bound syndromes 132

delirium 127
  psychopathology 94, 103
delusions 80, 101
delusional disorder 95
dementia 116
  drug treatment 71
  progression 113
  syndromes 140
depersonalization 97
depression
  psychodynamics 109
  psychopathology 82
development
  neurodevelopment 37
  stages 26
disorders of consciousness 104
drug interactions 69

electroencephalogram 149
emotion 23, 36
endocrine disorders 124, 142

formal thought disorder 85

gender development 18
generalized anxiety disorder 98
Goffman 19

hallucinations
  auditory 102
  experiences 92

ICD-10
  diagnosis 111
  hierarchy 128
  psychotic disorders 146

language development 14
learning theory 10, 17
  operant conditioning 1, 6
lobar functions 7

memory 34
mood disorders in DSM-IV 136
mood disturbances 78, 93
mood stabilizers 44
  anticonvulsants 65
  lithium 61, 74
  pharmacodynamics 67
moral development 13, 29
motivation 3
movement disorders 81, 145
multiple sclerosis 147

neuropsychiatry syndromes 8

object relations 108
old age disorders 123

panic disorder 87
paraphilias 121
perception 5, 30
  disorders 105
  sensory distortions 91

visual 20
personality assessment 24
personality disorders
  behaviour 125
  DSM-IV 129, 138
pharmacokinetics 42, 51
phenotypic similarities 150
physical signs 122
Piaget 2, 11
prejudice 25
problem-solving 16
psychiatric interview 110, 114
psychodynamics
  defence mechanisms 75, 79, 107
  theorists 76, 96, 100
psychological testing 31
psychopathology
  German 89
  syndromes 77
psychotherapy 134, 135
puerperium
  depression 133
  psychotropic use 49, 54

schizophrenia 115
  concepts 112
  first-rank symptoms 88
  outcome 143
  paranoid subtype 99
  psychopathology 86
social causation 119
self-concept 27
sleep disorders 126, 130
social influence 38
somatoform disorders 120
speech disorders 90
substance misuse treatment 56

vitamin deficiencies 148